BREAKING
THE
STRONGHOLD
OF
FOOD

BREAKING
THE
STRONGHOLD
OF
FOOD

MICHAEL L. BROWN
WITH NANCY BROWN

SILOAM

Most CHARISMA HOUSE BOOK GROUP products are available at special quantity discounts for bulk purchase for sales promotions, premiums, fund-raising, and educational needs. For details, write Charisma House Book Group, 600 Rinehart Road, Lake Mary, Florida 32746, or telephone (407) 333-0600.

BREAKING THE STRONGHOLD OF FOOD by Michael L. Brown, PhD
  with Nancy Brown
Published by Siloam
Charisma Media/Charisma House Book Group
600 Rinehart Road
Lake Mary, Florida 32746
www.charismahouse.com

Cover design by Lisa Rae McClure
Design Director: Justin Evans

Visit the author's website at www.AskDrBrown.org.

Library of Congress Cataloging-in-Publication Data:

Names: Brown, Michael L., 1955- author. | Brown, Nancy, 1954- author.
Title: Breaking the stronghold of food : how we conquered food addictions and
   discovered a new way of living / Michael L. Brown, PhD with Nancy Brown.
Description: Lake Mary, Florida : Siloam, [2017]
Identifiers: LCCN 2016045500| ISBN 9781629990996 (paperback) | ISBN
   9781629991009 (ebook)
Subjects: LCSH: Compulsive eating--Psychological aspects. | Compulsive
   eaters--Rehabilitation. | Compulsive eating--Religious aspects. |
   Obesity--Humor. | BISAC: RELIGION / Christian Life / Personal Growth. |
   HEALTH & FITNESS / Healthy Living.
Classification: LCC RC552.C65 B76 2017 | DDC 616.85/26--dc23
LC record available at https://lccn.loc.gov/2016045500

17 18 19 20 21 — 9 8 7 6 5 4 3 2 1
Printed in the United States of America

CONTENTS

PREFACE

T HIS IS THE first book Nancy and I have written together, and we are excited and amazed. We're excited because it's our first joint effort of this kind after being together since 1974 and sharing so much in life and ministry. We're amazed because, until the last few years, we've been anything but a poster couple for healthy eating habits. Quite the contrary! But that's part of what makes this book so special. As we say many times in the pages that follow, if we can make these radical, liberating changes, so can you.

In this book I'll tell the story of my own life transformation, incorporating many spiritual lessons and practical guidelines along the way. Nancy read every word of my portion of the book carefully, massively improving the contents. Then, whenever she saw fit, she added her own thoughts—in my opinion, her words are worth their weight in gold—so you'll find them throughout the book. Then, in appendix A, you can read her own story from beginning to end. We trust you will be encouraged, edified, blessed, and challenged, and we pray that the Lord will use this book to help you transform your own life as well.

Nancy and I want to make clear that this is not a medical book, not a nutritional book, not a diet book, and not a recipe book. It is a book that, by God's grace, will help you break the stronghold of food in your life and lead you into a whole new way of living and eating. Whatever sacrifices this entails, those sacrifices will absolutely be worth it, without a doubt. Living self-controlled lives as good stewards of our bodies is certainly God's will, and we know that God's will is best and that His ways are ways of life—abundant life!

Throughout the book, we will encourage you to stop eating unhealthy foods and to start eating healthy foods. But to repeat: this is neither a medical nor a nutritional book. I am the last one to offer professional medical advice—my doctorate is in Near Eastern Languages and Literatures, and I am more equipped to discuss the ancient Semitic vocabulary for the word *doctor* than to give you medical advice. As for Nancy, although she has studied nutrition for several decades, she is not a professional nutritionist, and so we refer you to other professionals. In appendix D we list recommended resources, including some recipe books.

In the book I make frequent mention of my workout routines—although you'll see that Nancy is not exactly an exercise fanatic—and so, with the goal of encouraging you in this area too, my trainer and I have put together a series of videos that you can follow. You can watch them for free at the Get Fit with Dr. Brown channel on YouTube.

Nancy and I really do understand how difficult it can be to break with a lifetime of bad eating habits, but we are sure it's the Lord's best plan that we do. And we're confident that if you put into practice the principles we lay out in this book, you can begin a whole new, wonderful chapter in your life. May Jesus be glorified in your body!

We want to express our appreciation to Adrienne Gaines and Debbie Marrie, key members of the Charisma Media team who helped make this book what it is. And lastly, on a personal note, I'm thrilled that my ministry audience can now be directly exposed to Nancy's wisdom. She has been a rock in my life for so many years, and I often speak of her influence when I preach and teach. Now you can hear her for yourself, which blesses me as much as I believe it will bless you.

Shall we begin?

CHAPTER 1

SET YOUR SIGHTS ON THE GOAL

L ET ME ENCOURAGE you to take your eyes off food for a moment and dream together with me, asking the simple question, "What if...?"

What if you could be the healthiest you've been in years (or maybe in your whole life), reversing some life-threatening diseases and finding yourself more vibrant at sixty than you were at forty, all without drugs?

What if you could be fit and trim, having tons more energy for your family, your friends, your job, your ministry, your hobbies, and your life, not to mention for your Lord?

What if you would never feel bloated or stuffed and never feel bad about what you ate?

What if you weren't ashamed of the way you look?

What if:

- Your stomach didn't sit on your lap.

- You could tie your shoes.

- You could see your toes.

- You could wear normal clothes rather than clothes that looked like tents.

- You didn't have to stealthily unbutton your pants at the restaurant (and remember to rebutton them when you got up to leave).

- You didn't have to wear stretchy pants.

- You didn't have to avoid mirrors (or plate glass windows).

- You didn't have to worry about buttons bursting off your shirt.

- You didn't have to buy all kinds of loose-fitting clothing to cover your fat.

- You didn't have to buy even bigger clothes the next year after the holidays and your latest weight gain.

What if? Only you know what bothers you most about your weight, and I write this not to shame you but to encourage you, since I too was once fat.

From Nancy: Some people might be offended by Mike's use of the word *fat*, but both of us like to tell it like it is. Many prefer to call it "overweight" (that certainly sounds more pleasant). But there was nothing pleasant or pretty about the fat on my body! So we will be using the words overweight and fat interchangeably throughout the book. But this is not meant to insult or criticize others. My fat was a hindrance to me and a burden that was choking and destroying my life. And the bottom line is, there was nothing nice or redeemable about the fat that encumbered my body.

What if you could do all this simply by changing your relationship to food? Would it be worth it? Would it be pleasing to the Lord? Would it enhance your witness and effectiveness? Would your loved ones appreciate it? Would *you* appreciate it?

The answer to these questions is obvious. Of course it would it be worth it. Of course it would be pleasing to the Lord; positive, not negative; good, not bad; for the better, not for the worse.

Then why do so many of us find ourselves overweight and obese, weighed down (literally) with food addictions, our energy sapped, our blood vessels clogged, our hearts overworked, our later years plagued with unnecessary disease? For the most part, it is because of our unhealthy relationship to unhealthy foods and, more specifically, because we don't know how to break free (or we're simply not willing to break free) from our bad habits.

I'm here to tell you that if Nancy and I could break free and change, you can too, with God's grace and help. I'm here to tell you that there is hope for your physical transformation. It's not a pipe dream. It's not hopeless and impossible. It's not too late, even if you have tried a thousand times, read the latest diet fad book, and taken the latest weight loss pill, all in vain.

In August of 2014 I weighed 275 pounds. Less than eight months later, after I began a new lifestyle of eating a healthy, plant-based diet, I weighed 180 pounds and had lost more than ten inches around my waist. I cannot tell you how wonderfully vibrant I feel!

From Nancy: In July 2012 I completely changed my lifestyle and started eating a healthy, plant-based diet. I did not weigh myself that first day—I didn't have the courage to get on the scale. A week later I finally weighed in at 195.5 pounds, so I'm quite sure I was over 200 pounds when I started. And I'm only 5 feet 2 inches! One year later, I was 114.5 pounds, which was less than I weighed in high school and, most likely, even junior high.

GETTING YOUNGER AND STRONGER

Recently, while ministering in Italy, I was talking with a colleague I've worked with there since 1987. He and I are about the same age, and we're watching our friends age along with us. He said to me, "You're the only one I know who's getting younger and stronger as you get older." That says it all!

Over the years my cholesterol has been as high as 240. Fifteen months after I began my lifestyle change, it was down to 123. My blood pressure got as high as 149/103. Today it averages 105/65. I used to get headaches two to three times a week. I have not had a headache in over two years.

For several years I battled a chronic cough, which was a real drag for me as a public speaker and talk-radio host. I saw several doctors and even a voice therapist, trying different medications and herbal solutions, without lasting success. About six months into this new lifestyle, I realized that the cough had disappeared. I can't tell you why; I just know it happened.

From Nancy: Most of the time I was in physical pain throughout my entire body. I didn't know exactly what was wrong and why I hurt so much, but I'm pretty sure that lugging around an extra 85 pounds every day of my life took its toll. Just try picking up an 85-pound dumbbell! (I don't even know that I could lift that much weight now, but I was forcing my body to do that every single day.) My joints hurt. My feet hurt. I just hurt— everywhere. I was exhausted all the time and had zero energy for even simple, everyday tasks. My cholesterol was up to 238 and my blood pressure was climbing, as were my glucose levels (all these had always been low before). The bigger issue for me, though, was the constant shame of wearing my overeating for all the world to see.

Almost fifteen years ago I was diagnosed with obstructive sleep apnea, meaning that I had to sleep with a breathing machine (called a CPAP machine; it forces a continual flow of air into your nose)—which meant that I had to travel with the machine wherever I went worldwide, taking it out for inspection when going through airport security (at airport after airport in country after country), trying to figure out how to use it on fifteen-hour overseas flights (where do you plug it in?). Oh yes, Dr. Michael Brown, the mighty man of God on his way to preach across the Atlantic, with the mask on his face, the blanket over his head, and the tube running into the machine. What a sight! And what do I tell the flight attendant when she comes by to make sure I'm OK?

The condition was getting worse, not better, to the point that it went from moderate to severe, meaning that without the breathing machine, my sleep was absolutely horrific, making my overseas trips much more difficult. So in addition to all the other challenges I faced, I was always sleep deprived.

Having sleep apnea also creates a vicious cycle of weight gain, since the worse your quality of sleep, the harder it is to lose weight, and the more weight you gain, the worse your sleep apnea becomes. By God's grace, the cycle has been broken in my life, and I no longer need to sleep with the machine. No more breathing machine! No more extra piece of carry-on luggage. No more trying to find an outlet near the bed in a small hotel in India. No more having to cover my head with a blanket while flying overseas. (From Nancy: And no more having our bedroom sound like a hospital room with someone on oxygen!) This is exclusively the result of weight loss.

Today not only has the sleep apnea been dealt with, but my immune system is radically stronger, something that is very important when you have a nonstop ministry lifestyle, with travel around the world, constantly moving from time zone to time zone and climate to climate. My energy level is off the charts, and sometimes I feel so light and free I just want to run—up the steps, into the grocery store, across the parking lot, everywhere. (Remember that I'm sixty-one years old as of this writing.) And miracle of miracles, this is all without energy drinks, special vitamins, or magic pills. (I have a whole chapter in the book about how much of a sucker I was for these energy-boosting and weight-loss products.)

From Nancy: There's something about getting down to your ideal weight. Something clicks in, and your body just feels amazing. There's a lightness, an airiness, an energy that's hard to articulate. Just as with Mike, all the physical heaviness disappeared. But it wasn't until I got all the way down to my ideal weight—when people said I was too thin—that I felt incredible. It's funny, we are so used to seeing people pudgy that we have lost sight of what a healthy person at a healthy weight actually looks like, which is why people told me I looked too thin.

My physical appearance now matches the way I have lived for decades—sold out to the Lord, living a Jesus-centered, countercultural lifestyle, saying no to the flesh and yes to God. Let me say it again: if I was able to make this radical change, with the Father's help, so can you.

What about the role of exercise in my life? Actually, for a good number of years, I exercised fairly regularly and quite intensively, to the point that much younger men couldn't keep up with me. Yet I was still overweight and eating a very unhealthy diet. My cholesterol was still too high (even though it had gone down from its highest point), and my blood pressure was reaching the early stages of hypertension. And here I was pushing myself to the limit, virtually to the point of collapse. Nancy kept warning me that it was unwise and even dangerous to exercise like that while eating the way I did.

Today when I exercise, I want to push myself even harder and my muscles recover much more quickly. But the reason I bring up exercise here is simple: all the exercise in the world can't take the place of changing your eating habits, and if you really want to be healthy and vibrant, you cannot escape the fact that you need to put good fuel into your body, not junky fuel. *The food you eat is the fuel.*

On a regular basis people ask me about the importance of exercise, and it certainly does play an important role. But if you had to pick between healthy eating and exercise, you must start with healthy eating. And then as you start to feel better, you'll be much more inclined to exercise because you won't be bogged down with exhaustion since you're no longer carrying around all that excess weight. So pick your battles carefully, and put your whole focus first on changing your eating habits.

From Nancy: Exercise—ugh! I have to admit that I'm not a big fan of formal exercise. I understand the importance of it and know it's a major key to a healthy lifestyle, but I find it to be a boring, mindless activity and something that I rarely enjoy. I do exercise on occasion, but I have to absolutely force myself. We've had the machines—a treadmill, a rowing machine, a stationary bike. We have videos and dumbbells, exercise bands, and weighted vests. And I just recently purchased yet another video (an exercise dance program that's not supposed to feel like exercise—they lied). So I know I should exercise, but truth be told, I usually don't. I'm still trying to learn to enjoy it, and I do attempt it once in a while. But I'm still in the process of conquering this.

On one occasion when I joined my husband and his trainer for some exercise, his trainer tried to push me as he does with all his clients. He did it in a very nice and gentle way, though. I explained to him that rather than the "no pain, no gain" philosophy most had, mine was, "When I feel the pain, I refrain." As soon as it gets hard, I stop. There's something about pushing my muscles to the point of the "burn" that just feels "wrong," uncomfortable, like having a finger stuck in your eyeball. I don't like it.

In any case, I was able to easily lose all the weight with little to no exercise, and even though I still don't participate in a formal exercise routine, my stamina has greatly increased. I do spend a lot of time outside gardening and moving my body. We live on seven acres, half of which is wooded, and you can find me there sawing down trees and branches and hauling the wood around, so I'm not totally a couch potato. But I'm still learning to enjoy exercise.

When it comes to food being your fuel, let me ask you a question. What would you think of a top NASCAR driver whose team spent millions of dollars fine-tuning his vehicle, yet he always finished last because he liked the smell of one particular fuel, even though it caused his car to run slowly? Wouldn't that be the height of folly? Well, if we want to be totally honest with ourselves, isn't it even more foolish to cut our lives short, to rob ourselves of energy and vitality, and to hinder our effectiveness for Jesus simply because we would rather eat ice cream, pizza, and french fries than salads, fruits, and beans?

The reality is that your palate will crave whatever you feed it so that over time you will enjoy healthy foods as much as you once enjoyed unhealthy foods. This was almost impossible for me to believe when both a doctor-friend and Nancy told me this years ago. No way! A bowl of fruit could never compare to a breakfast of Oreos, and a spinach salad could never hit the spot at midnight like jelly beans and peanut M&Ms.

The truth be told, not only did I not believe that I could ever change my palate, but I had no desire to change my palate. I thoroughly enjoyed unhealthy eating, and it's all I knew my entire life. And every year for the holidays and my birthday, my family and friends gave me every kind of sweet treat wrapped up in the most beautiful paper. Even the graduating class of my ministry school once gave me a special gift of sweets. And when I traveled to preach, chocolates and sweets were always waiting in the gift basket in my hotel rooms while in every airport I knew where to get my favorite treats. (There are a *lot* of airports around the world!)

Today, when I walk through the grocery store, I crave apples. I can't wait to have fresh fruit in the morning in my hotel room, and I absolutely look forward to my massive, super-healthy salad every night. *I promise you: your taste buds will change if you give them a chance.* It just takes time.

From Nancy: This was a biggie for me. I do not naturally crave broccoli or apples or healthy foods in general (fruits and vegetables). I do not gravitate toward them. I would much rather have piles of pasta with gobs of a buttery, cheesy, creamy sauce and a bag of Lindt chocolate truffles. When I started eating healthfully, I absolutely despised the new food. It made me nauseated. I literally felt like I was going to vomit.

I actually thought to myself, "I'm going to have to quit because I just cannot do this." But I knew that my health was at stake and I was eating myself to death.

So that's the thing that drove me. I pressed on, and I tried to have a positive attitude. I shopped for the healthiest foods, and I tried new recipes, cooking like a mad woman.

On my very first attempt at preparing something healthy, I made a huge pot of vegetable soup using a well-tested recipe I had discovered online. I cooked it in the biggest pot I had—it was enough for a small army—and I couldn't wait to try it. But when I had my first spoonful, I was shocked to find it tasted so horrid I just couldn't get it down. I didn't have the heart to throw it away, so I divided it into individual servings and put them in the freezer (not actually having a clue what I was going to do with them).

Some months later, after my taste buds had truly changed, I defrosted one of the servings and had a bowl of the soup—it was absolutely scrumptious. I devoured it. Truly a miracle in my eyes! And it proves the point that we're making here: If you genuinely want to eat healthy things and have never been able to eat them before, you can train yourself. Your taste buds will change. Guaranteed. It just takes a little time and effort.

Most of the time, when we taste something new and we don't like it, that particular food gets added to our "Do not eat" list, never to be tried again. But if we know it's good for our bodies, and we are determined to change our eating style, we can overcome the taste bud issue. We just have to be willing to push ourselves a bit. I was absolutely convinced that I could never learn to like food that I, well, didn't like. I was told just what I'm telling you here—that it's possible to change. But I believed I was the exception to the rule. As it turns out, I'm not an exception at all. I have put in the effort to train myself, and the training was successful. It can be done. Things that I literally gagged on (such as mushrooms), I now eat and actually enjoy. But it took practice, determination, and trying over and over again to get to the point where my palate changed. So, how important is it to you to gain your health and life back? How badly do you want it?

What stops you, then, from making a life-changing transition? Is it ignorance? Lack of willingness? The power of food addictions? Lack of time?

I LOVE MY FOOD...

Consider this scenario. Your doctor says to you, "You don't have to be on medication for high blood pressure and cholesterol, you can avoid serious and invasive heart surgery, you can be cured of your type 2 diabetes, you can add years of health and vitality to your life, and you can have so much more energy for your family, friends, job, and ministry work."

You say in reply, "I know it's true, but I love my food."

Is this an acceptable answer for a believer? Would it be acceptable in any other area of life? Would we ever say, "Yes, Lord, I know Your will, but I love my pornography (or adultery or violence or stealing or gambling or drunkenness or gossip)"?

Obviously, there's nothing inherently sinful about food itself, but at the very least, we should recognize that food addiction and bad eating habits can be powerful strongholds in our lives—they certainly were in my life for decades—and if they are controlling us, we should confess this to the Lord. Acknowledging the problem is the first step to solving the problem.

One Christian leader once said, "Make it your habit to have no habits." I would quote that to others and then say to myself, "But you have your habits. You're addicted to chocolate and pizza and other foods. You're not free." I recognized the problem and realized that these habits were potentially deadly, but I wasn't willing to do anything about it.

Honestly, making changes in my diet seemed like an utter impossibility. Plus, I thought to myself, everybody eats like this anyway. It's the normal American lifestyle. Why should I be the one eating lettuce leaves when everyone else is feasting?

For many years I had my list of excuses, and to me they were quite compelling. (Isn't it funny that when someone else makes the same excuses you do, those excuses sound so weak and wimpy? We'll take this up again in chapter 13.) I was so bound by certain food addictions and mental strongholds that even when I had a bad cold and couldn't taste, I would *still* eat unhealthy foods. (Sound familiar?) To say it once more: if I could make this radical lifestyle change, you can too, especially if you have the Lord in your life.

From Nancy: I never, ever once thought for a moment that I had an addiction. I'm a strong individual, and I consider myself mentally tough and always assumed that nothing really had power over me, which begs the question: How did I get to 200 pounds, all the time knowing that it was extremely detrimental to my health? And why was I unable to get that weight off?

It wasn't until I was well on my journey of healthful eating that I realized the pull food had on me. Even in the beginning, when I felt I couldn't make the change, it didn't dawn on me that I was addicted. Sometimes we can be so blind to our own weaknesses. The real clincher for me was when I was well within reach of my weight goal, and I allowed myself a little cheat here and there, just a little something forbidden (unhealthy). It started out as a minor, once-a-month splurge. The timing was always controlled and planned out and never a spur-of-the-moment temptation I yielded to. This worked for a little while, but eventually, each time I indulged in my splurge, the very next day I had zero desire for all the healthy foods I had come to enjoy. And one splurge day became two and then three (you get the picture).

It opened up the floodgates of almost uncontrollable cravings. Just as an alcoholic cannot have a sip of alcohol, as a food addict there was no such thing as moderation for me. There was no such thing as a little taste or bite. That would open Pandora's box. You hear many people say, "Everything in moderation." But to the addict, moderation is not a possibility. Now that might not be the case for everyone. Some people can have a little taste now and then of certain "treats" and they're fine. It doesn't thrust them into a binge. But that just does not work for me. I know my limitations, and my past behaviors bear it out. It's extremely important to be able to pinpoint your weaknesses and adjust your lifestyle accordingly. If eating a bit of a chocolate cake has the potential to cause you to eat the entire bakery boxful, it's pretty clear there is a problem.

Yes, food strongholds are powerful, but isn't the power of the Spirit greater than the power of doughnuts? Isn't the life of Jesus inside of you—the life of the resurrected Son of God—greater than any food addiction? When God says you are an overcomer in Him, yes, even more than a conqueror, doesn't that include victory over potato chips?

I'm not talking about some kind of dieting gimmick or fad. I'm talking about transforming your life and totally changing how you relate to food. I'm talking about being a disciple when it comes to eating, about taking on a whole new way of living—a wonderful way. And the great thing about it is that when you make the change and renew your mind and reprogram your habits, you won't feel deprived at all. You'll thrive.

Nancy and I are living witnesses to it, and you can be too. So what stops you from taking the plunge?

From Nancy: What a wonderful feeling it is to have the guilt removed from your eating and to know that you're pleasing the Lord with your lifestyle. There's a cloud that lifts off. I wasn't always consciously aware of this, but there was a constant, underlying tension that I felt all the time. Interestingly, I wasn't fully aware of this until it went away and I felt so free (as a result of eating healthily).

Why not take a moment and prayerfully write down what stops you from making a radical change in your eating habits: fear that you won't be able to do it; love of certain foods; intense dislike of wholesome foods; food addictions; lack of desire to change; lack of money to buy healthy foods; not knowing what to do next; the seeming impossibility of maintaining a healthy lifestyle; juggling the needs of your family and your schedule; lack of faith that you could ever change; lack of confidence that anything we're presenting in this book will work. Whatever the reasons may be, write them down and present them before your Father and say, "Lord, I'm weak! I need Your help! But I do want to change. Manifest Your grace in me and empower me to do Your will." I tell you again: if He did it for us, He'll do it for you.

I am *sure* the changes in our lives did not happen simply because of Nancy's amazing—and I do mean amazing—willingness to learn a new, better way of eating, or because of the willpower we exerted. God intervened and helped us. He'll help you too.

From Nancy: I really devoted myself to praying for Mike—I mean heartfelt, fighting, persistent praying—prayer that prays through, the type of prayer that knows it has to obtain the answer. I knew that, naturally speaking, this change was a complete impossibility for him. He was so set in his ways and had such a limited palate. That coupled with his traveling, the excuses he always made, and the amount of weight he had to lose—I knew it was impossible in the natural. Although Mike was always eager to try the newest energy pill or herbal, miracle fat buster, he was not the type to always be on a "diet," and the idea of making a sincere dietary change was truly a foreign thing (unlike many of us ladies who are always dieting). God absolutely poured out His grace on him.

God will pour out His grace on you, but you must realize how crucial the issue is in order to make a serious, lasting change. For me, being overweight was draining my energy and potentially cutting short my life, yet it didn't stop me from living a normal, active, and very productive life. But for many of you, being overweight has totally dominated your life: it has robbed you of normal relationships; it has stolen your confidence and caused you to hide yourself away because you're ashamed to be in public; it has stopped you from functioning as the parent or spouse or employee or friend or family member or minister that you're called to be; it has permeated every area of your life and hindered everything you do.

From Nancy: What can I say? That describes me to a tee. I despised being overweight. It was a gigantic cloud over my entire life. It was a stronghold beyond all strongholds. It was *the* stronghold. It permeated everything, controlled everything, and affected everything. It dominated my entire life—and really, I had no life since I rarely left the house. I had removed myself from social functions because I was just too ashamed of the way I looked. My life was on hold. I was eating enormous quantities of food and just felt sick all the time. Some of you can totally relate to what I'm saying here. For others, though, while your situation is not as extreme, being overweight is still an underlying, constant hindrance in your life. You're perpetually on a diet, you always hate the way you look, and you're always dissatisfied with where you're at because of your weight. Certainly that's no way to live and is not God's design for us.

The good news is that you are not doomed to die without victory over food, and there is definitely a way out for you. There is a place of freedom, health, and vitality and a whole new life that is hard to imagine from your vantage point of being so weighed down.

That's why we have written this book: to give you hope, confidence, motivation, and a vision for a brand-new, incredibly blessed life. It excites us as we write these words!

QUESTIONS FOR REFLECTION

1. Do I love my food more than I love my health, my family, or my Lord?

2. Is food a genuine stronghold in my life?

3. Do I believe that, with God's help, I can change my relationship to food and break the stronghold of food?

4. If the Lord is calling me to make a change— or if my health or just common sense calls for a change—am I willing to make sacrifices to see that change come?

CHAPTER 2

CONFESSIONS OF A RECOVERING FOOD ADDICT

W HEN THE LORD set me free from shooting drugs on December 17, 1971, at the age of sixteen, I was really set free. Totally free. I never put a needle in my arm again after that night. Two days later I swore off all other drugs, and by God's grace that was the end of the story. Drugs had no part in my life, and the more I walked with the Lord, the less interest I had in ever going back to my old, sinful ways. Jesus really delivered me.

Because of that, I could never relate to anyone who said, "I'm a recovering alcoholic," or, "I'm a recovering drug addict." Not me! That is who I *was*. It is not who I am today.

But when it comes to food—which all of us eat every day and which, in many unhealthy ways, was a major part of my life for my first sixty years—I consider myself a recovering food addict. Yet it is not because I'm tempted day and night or because I'm not committed to a healthy lifestyle. Actually,

I'm thriving, enjoying the blessings of God, thrilled to be thin and fit, and genuinely enjoying wholesome eating.

It's just that I realize that food is around us all the time, that many have started on this path and after short-term progress experienced long-term failure, and that I could fail as easily as anyone else did—"there go I but by the grace of God." And while there was no good reason for me ever to have contact with the drug world again, all of us are constantly in the food world. And since I'm constantly on the road, traveling throughout America and around the world, my attitude is like that of a recovering alcoholic who thinks to himself, "Just one sip, and I could fall back."

Do I believe that's the case at this stage of my life? I sure hope not! But I don't plan to find out.

For me, the only way to guarantee that I don't fall back into my old, unhealthy lifestyle is to keep the door closed against it, and I mean closed. Completely closed. Locked and shuttered. In other words, I'm done for life with being a poor steward of my body, but I say this in deep dependence on the Lord rather than in an attitude of presumption. The longer I live a healthy, God-glorifying lifestyle, the more wonderful it is, the greater the benefits, and the easier it becomes since the bad stuff just doesn't tempt me and the good stuff tastes better and better. (Plus in all likelihood, if I have some of the old foods after months and months of healthy eating, I'd probably get really sick.)

In this book, we want to do our best to encourage you to make a radical change in your own life, sharing our own stories since, *if we could make this change, anyone could.*

It's not because I was a glutton, although I was definitely a slave to unhealthy foods.

It's not because I was totally undisciplined in my life, although in the area of fast food or sweets or non-nutritious snacks, I indulged myself daily.

It's not because I didn't work out or push myself physically, although I virtually ignored the advice of my trainer who said, "Abs are made in the kitchen."

My problem was that I was a food wimp with unhealthy eating habits my entire life. And so, over the years, I got heavier and heavier, despite my rigorous schedule and despite really intense workouts. Little by little, my blood pressure was going up, my cholesterol remained too high, and I was getting more and more tired, especially with the day-and-night ministry schedule I kept.

From Nancy: It was very different for me. I was a glutton. It sounds terrible, doesn't it? But it's the truth. I normally ate whatever I wanted in enormous quantities, and that certainly didn't include fruits and vegetables. I loved highly processed, fatty, salty foods; pastas; cheeses; cream sauces; and, of course, gooey chocolate desserts. And I would eat until I was completely stuffed and uncomfortable—literally. Isn't that being a glutton? And isn't that the height of being undisciplined, to be eating that way when you know you shouldn't and you know it's killing you? I was not a food wimp like Mike. I would try anything and liked a lot of different foods. But what's interesting is that I was never gluttonous with broccoli or peaches or other healthy foods. It was only the highly processed, sugary, salty foods that drove me to overeat. Green beans were self-limiting.

Of course, I knew that if I ate differently, I would be much healthier, my physical appearance would be more God-glorifying (can you imagine Jesus being obese?), and I would be a better steward over my body, allowing me to serve God more effectively as I entered my sixties. Still, there was no way I could make such a radical change in my diet—at least, that's what I thought. It simply wouldn't work, and I knew it. The only dietary changes I ever made were for periods of months (or maybe a year), but even then they addressed only part of the problem, namely, eating less of the bad foods. They never addressed the other part of the problem: I simply did not eat lots of truly healthy food.

Fruit? Almost never, except for some occasional watermelon when I was trying to be "good." Apples? I used to eat them every so often—maybe once a year—but I became allergic to them (really, because of pollen). Oranges? Nope. Cantaloupe? Pineapple? Strawberries? Raspberries? Blueberries? Blackberries? Pears? Honeydew? (And on and on the list goes.) Nope. Not once. I never even tasted most of them. Why? Because I said, "I don't like them." (That was my code for, "I've never tasted them, and I don't plan to.") In fact, when Nancy would ask me to pick up fruit at the store, she often had to tell me what they looked like so I could spot them.

Vegetables? Well, I had a small salad virtually every day, and I really enjoyed it, but it was always with unhealthy dressing and with very limited items. As for things like brussels sprouts, I tried eating one of them years ago and literally almost choked on it. I had to spit it out. Yuck! Kale? Not a chance! Beans? No way!

It just seemed the healthier something was, the less I liked it, to the point that I virtually never tried eating new foods. Many times I told colleagues overseas that I would rather preach to an angry, potentially violent crowd than taste new foods, and they are my witnesses that I lived those words out.

What about breads? Bring them on! At Olive Garden I could easily eat four breadsticks (or more). Red Lobster? Those biscuits were the best! Keep bringing them out from the kitchen, and I'll keep eating them. Even at a cheap buffet like Golden Corral, I'd down a bunch of those yeast rolls with butter.

What about pizza and pasta? Suffice it to say that I could have gladly lived on pizza and pasta the rest of my life—actually, just on pizza (and I mean the real deal pizza, New York style or the like)—and I would have been perfectly content with the same meal every day. In fact, while teaching at a Bible school on Long Island from 1983 to 1987, I estimate that I ate three thousand slices of pizza at an incredible pizzeria just two miles from the school during those years. The slices there were dripping in cheese—over the years I never found another place quite like it—and I was there so frequently that I actually had an account where I had to pay only once a month.

I NEVER MET A PIECE OF CHOCOLATE I DIDN'T LIKE...

What about sweets? Now you're talking! I was a confirmed chocoholic, definitely addicted to chocolate and other sweets for most of my life. My son-in-law Ryan told me that he never saw anyone enjoy chocolate as much I did, and his family bought me a T-shirt that said, "I never met a piece of chocolate that I didn't like."

After a meal, I would crave sweets, and as much as I enjoyed eating my daily candy bar or ice cream or M&Ms or whatever it was, I actually needed to have them to satisfy that craving. But what do you expect from someone who used to eat Oreo cookies for breakfast as a boy? (As you can probably tell, I did not grow up in a household that emphasized healthy, nutritional eating.) When I'd check in at a hotel and there were fresh-baked chocolate chip cookies on the counter, I would always grab a couple (or three), and if there was a welcome basket with chocolates in my room, most of them would be gone the same night.

One time in the early 1980s I went to a diner with some friends after a meeting and ordered a chocolate milkshake and two brownies. One of my friends, who, like me, used to shoot drugs, said to me, "Why don't you just shoot it in your veins?" That's how much I liked chocolate.

I also have an addictive personality, so I thrive on doing more and pushing harder, which can be fruitful and productive when channeled in the right direction for the right purpose. But it's totally destructive in other ways, as I saw with my drug use as a teenager. What satisfied me yesterday didn't satisfy me today. I needed more.

It was the same thing with food, and although I had eaten pretty much the same way for years, in the year leading up to my radical lifestyle change, I began to see this same addictive problem creeping in with foods. The two big slices of New York pizza that satisfied me before didn't really do it anymore. When it came to ice cream, a big dish of chocolate ice cream was no longer enough. I needed a pint of Ben & Jerry's New York Super Fudge Chunk chocolate ice cream. Or I needed a large Chocolate Extreme Dairy Queen Blizzard (even as I type those words, I remember how I used to savor that Blizzard, sometimes skipping a meal to justify eating it, since it had 1,380 calories, including 37 grams of saturated fat, about double what someone should have in an entire day). And if I did have just a bowl of regular chocolate ice cream, I would have to heap on the chocolate syrup to hit the spot.

This led to the obvious question: "What next?" What is there beyond the most decadent ice cream treats available? (Oh yes, there was actually a new Dove ice cream that was just about as decadent—and as deadly—so that also worked for a special treat every so often.)

But, to repeat, I was not a glutton in terms of being out of control with my overall diet. In the morning (normally mid- to late morning because of my late-night schedule), I would have a big chocolate protein bar (convinced that it was healthy because of the protein, although Nancy would always tell me it was not). Then I'd skip lunch, have a slice or two of pizza or some pasta for dinner, always with a small salad, then something chocolate for dessert. Then I'd snack at night continually as I sat at the computer and wrote into the early hours of the morning (some pretzel sticks, some jelly beans, some more pretzel sticks, some more jelly beans, another piece of chocolate—you get the picture).

But I would not just pig out. For the most part I avoided fried foods and didn't eat that much red meat (I'd eat it maybe a couple times a month), although I loved a good burger and would thoroughly enjoy going to a nice steak house on special occasions. I normally avoided McDonald's and the like (or, if I did eat there, I would often get a grilled chicken sandwich since it was "healthier" than the other stuff—but with fries, of course; that being said, I had more than my share of chicken nuggets). Sometimes I would have ice cream every day for most of a week and then not have it for weeks after that. Every day I would say no to certain foods I wanted to eat. And often, because of ministry and travel, I would miss meals and have to do without. No problem at all.

Yet I was obese, my clothes were getting tighter—I mean my "fat" clothes, the ones that were supposed to be loose fitting—and I was increasingly embarrassed by my weight, feeling that the way I looked didn't reflect the way I lived. In one sense I was a disciplined servant of the Lord and a leader with a very public ministry, but in another sense I indulged the flesh every day and I looked quite slovenly, to say the least.

Looking back at before-and-after pictures now, I'm flabbergasted and terribly embarrassed to see how fat I was. Interestingly, many others say to me now, "I don't ever remember you being that heavy." *I was*. Pictures don't lie, nor does the scale.

From Nancy: If there was one thing that was the straw that broke the camel's back for me—the thing that caused me to change my lifestyle—it was that I was starting to feel really sick, physically sick. There was pain throughout my entire body, and I didn't know what was wrong with me. I thought I could be seriously ill, and I knew I was doing nothing to prevent disease on my own. God is full of grace and mercy, but He is not obligated to keep us healthy while we're abusing our bodies. We do reap what we sow. It's a biblical principle, and it applies all the more when we know we're doing wrong. How would I ever be able to pray for health with genuine faith while I did not have a clear conscience about what I was inflicting on my body—the body the Lord owned? If our consciences are not clear before the Lord, we are conflicted, and it is impossible to pray in faith in that state, and I knew that. To find out what steps I took to break the stronghold of food in my life, see appendix B.

But what was I to do? There was absolutely no way I could make a lasting, radical change (or so I thought), first because I didn't like almost all the foods I would need to eat, and second because my travel schedule made it impossible. I had watched Nancy transform her life through healthy eating, but it took time to prepare the meals and she needed to buy certain ingredients (in contrast, eating fast food is as easy as it is deadly).

What was I going to do during my annual trip to India? What was I going to eat on fifteen-hour flights? What about the endless days spent at hotels? What about the countless meals at restaurants before or after preaching?

What I learned is that all these obstacles can be overcome, and if I can make a lasting change like this, anyone can. By God's grace (a phrase I use a lot, especially in this book), it is totally possible. And soon enough, if you take the plunge, you'll be as amazed at the brand-new life you're living, just as I have been amazed at the new life I am living.

Are you ready to take another step in the right direction? Then turn the page.

QUESTIONS FOR REFLECTION

1. Do you have food addictions? If so, what are they? Confess them to the Lord as sinful and destructive.

2. What are your bad eating habits? What are your good eating habits?

3. What embarrasses you most about being overweight?

4. What one thing scares you the most about making a lifestyle change? Share this openly with the Lord. He already knows!

CHAPTER 3

WHAT IF UNHEALTHY EATING IS SINFUL?

A RE WE "DIGGING our own graves with forks and knives," as a leading doctor claims?[1] A new study "reveals that obesity is linked to very high rates of chronic illnesses— higher than living in poverty, and much higher than smoking or drinking."[2] Have we adequately considered the health risks of obesity, not to mention the spiritual side of obesity?

I do not want to lay a guilt trip on anyone, and if you are overweight or aware that your diet is unhealthy, you probably feel bad enough already. So the last thing I want to do is make you feel even worse. Instead, I want to talk with you heart-to-heart, encouraging you to consider whether there might be a serious spiritual dimension to unhealthy eating. This could be the incentive you need to make a positive change.

Let's think about drunkenness for a moment. As followers of Jesus we know that getting drunk is sinful in God's sight. It impairs us in many ways, and it is life destroying in many ways. And so long-term alcoholism can be deadly, not only because of the dangers of drunk driving or the possibilities of unwise behavior while drunk but also because of cirrhosis of the liver and other diseases. If we abuse our bodies with alcohol, there will be consequences.

How about cigarette smoking? I imagine most believers feel this is sinful as well. The question is: Why? Is it dangerous to smoke while driving? Not in a major way. Does smoking cigarettes impair our judgment and twist our behavior the way drunkenness does? Certainly not. Then why do we believe it is wrong? Aside from being a wasteful addiction, the obvious answer is that it is destructive to our bodies, leading to lung cancer and other deadly conditions.

What about unhealthy eating, which can mean eating in excess (gluttony) or eating the wrong foods? (Often, it is a combination of both.) Is that sinful in God's sight? In most cases, unhealthy eating causes us to be overweight, and Dr. Joel Fuhrman, whom I will cite frequently in this book, lists the following as health risks of obesity:

- Increased overall premature mortality

- Adult-onset diabetes

- Hypertension

- Degenerative arthritis

- Coronary artery disease

- Cancer

- Lipid disorders

- Obstructive sleep apnea

- Gallstones

- Fatty infiltration of liver

- Restrictive lung disease

- Gastrointestinal diseases[3]

Dr. Fuhrman describes this in a chapter titled "Digging Our Graves with Forks and Knives," and he is not exaggerating. Would we, as God's children, knowingly engage in any other behavior that had such deadly consequences and did such harm to our bodies? Would we smoke and drink and do drugs, knowing the dangers involved, and say, "It's no big deal; the Lord understands"? Not if we were serious about following Him.

Then why do we have such a different attitude when it comes to food, even when there is no denying our obesity and our lack of discipline? Why is this the acceptable destructive practice? Even when unhealthy eating does not lead to obesity, it still leads to serious long-term health problems. Why, then, do we say so little about it?

A respected surgeon and health expert in England recently commented that "the obesity epidemic was as bad for public health as the 1919 flu epidemic."[4] How bad was that epidemic? According to History.com, "The influenza or flu pandemic of 1918 to 1919, the deadliest in modern history, infected an estimated 500 million people worldwide—about one-third of the planet's population at the time—and killed an estimated 20 million to 50 million victims. More than 25 percent of the U.S. population became sick, and some 675,000 Americans died during the pandemic."[5] And this British expert is comparing this deadly flu epidemic to today's obesity epidemic. Do we just ignore this and go on with our blissful (and destructive) lifestyles?

Again, I don't want to embarrass anyone, but something is wrong when there is so much obesity in our midst (meaning, within the church). Something is wrong when so many of our leaders are grossly overweight—and I say that with the utmost sympathy, wanting only to help, not to hurt. (I was one of those grossly overweight leaders!) Perhaps here and there, someone has a genuine metabolic disorder or a thyroid issue or the like, and their weight gain has little to do with their lifestyle. But that person is extremely rare, to put it mildly. The vast majority of our obesity is due either to gluttony and/or unhealthy eating. Lack of exercise certainly factors in as well, but I was living proof that you could work out heavily, pushing your cardio to the limit, and still be seriously overweight.

The problem with unhealthy eating is that it's not as easily recognized as, say, watching pornography, getting drunk, or losing your temper and putting your fist through a wall. We all eat every day, normally several times a day, and most of us don't think that having a big steak one night is sinful or that we're in disobedience to God if we have an ice cream cone at a birthday party. And I'm not saying it is sinful to do this every so often, nor am I your judge or spiritual policeman.

Many of us eat out at restaurants on a regular basis, but the average menu in the average restaurant is filled with unhealthy foods (or the foods are prepared in unhealthy ways), and the portions are often enormous. I'm constantly taken out for meals when I'm on the road, and it was also my habit for decades to eat out at least one time a day when I was home. Even exercising restraint at every meal, almost never eating as much of whatever I wanted (even at an all-you-can-eat buffet), there's no question that eating like this is unhealthy, even though it seems perfectly normal in our culture.

Does this sound familiar? "Let's share some of that cheese bread for an appetizer, OK? Or should we get those new pretzel sticks with dipping sauce? Or maybe the spicy chicken wings? How about a big sampler of our favorite four appetizers? Yeah, let's do that. And we'll tell the server to bring out some extra rolls. They have the best rolls here!"

Before we know it, even without the main course and, yes, even without that massive dessert, we have already had more than enough unhealthy calories for the whole day, not to mention increased our addiction to unhealthy foods. And even if this is not a daily or weekly habit, most of the foods we tend to eat at home are loaded with unhealthy content although we're largely unaware of it.

What we *are* aware of is our gradual weight gain or the gradual deterioration of our health. And so, over the course of time, if we see that we are putting on weight or our blood pressure is rising or we are developing other health conditions—such as back problems or knee problems that are caused by being overweight—then we have to stop and ask ourselves, "What am I doing wrong?" God has designed our bodies with incredible wisdom, far beyond our understanding, and He has made them to function wonderfully. Why are we putting substandard and even destructive fuel into this incredible, living mechanism?

Over the years, as I was getting older and my diet was still unhealthy, I often reflected on this very thing: Despite putting subpar fuel into my body almost all of my life, it was still functioning well—really, it was functioning very well—and I was profoundly grateful for that. But wasn't I abusing my Father's grace? (If you're reading this book and you don't even believe in God, think in terms of pushing your luck.)

I'd think to myself, "What would happen if I ate well? How would my body respond then?" I'd also think to myself, "My heart has only so many beats. Why cut my life short by putting extra pressure on it, making it carry around all this extra weight? Isn't this sinning against God and my family, not to mention against those the Lord has called me to minister to?" I also understood that layers of fat around my stomach are often a precursor to cancer and heart disease. Why would I even allow for these deadly possibilities?

Now that I'm thin, my trainer will sometimes have me work out wearing a twenty-pound vest, and it feels like a whole lot more than that, especially when I'm putting it on. Just try running up and down the stairs ten times carrying that extra weight, let alone doing pushups, burpees, and jump squats. Clearly, you are putting extra stress on your whole body when you do that, and we're only talking about an extra twenty pounds. What about that extra ninety-five pounds I used to carry? And what about doing it all the time as opposed to doing it just for the purpose of exercise? Why are we putting so much extra stress on our bodies?

OUR BODIES ARE NOT OUR OWN

But there's something more, and I want you to take a moment to reflect on this before the Lord: *Your body is not your own*. It does not belong to you; it belongs to the Lord. This means that, just as you are a steward of your finances, you are a steward of your body. How are you taking care of this extraordinarily valuable piece of property that is owned by the Lord and has been entrusted to you? How are you taking care of your health?

Along with your relationship with the Lord and your loved ones, your health is one of the most important things in your life. After all, if your health is shot—if you are constantly sick or unable to function normally or if you die prematurely—neither your money nor your good reputation nor your family and friends can help you. But there's also the spiritual dimension to your health. To the extent your health depends on you, you are accountable to God.

Although Paul was writing to the Corinthians about the dangers of sexual immorality, it is not a stretch to make a larger application of his counsel. He wrote, "Flee from sexual immorality. Every other sin a person commits is outside the body, but the sexually immoral person sins against his own body. Or do you not know that your body is a temple of the Holy Spirit within you, whom you have from God? You are not your own, for you were bought with a price. So glorify God in your body" (1 Cor. 6:18–20).

So, even though the emphasis here is on sexual purity, if 1) our bodies are not our own, 2) our bodies are temples of the Holy Spirit, and 3) we are called to glorify God in our bodies, can we truly do this if we are abusing our bodies? If we are gradually destroying our bodies? If we are displaying a serious lack of discipline in what we put into our bodies?

Later in 1 Corinthians, Paul wrote this:

> Do you not know that in a race all the runners run, but only one receives the prize? So run that you may obtain it. Every athlete exercises self-control in all things. They do it to receive a perishable wreath, but we an imperishable. So I do not run aimlessly; I do not box as one beating the air. But I discipline my body and keep it under control, lest after preaching to others I myself should be disqualified.
>
> —1 Corinthians 9:24–27

Notice carefully what Paul is saying since we often miss an important point in this passage. Paul is urging us to run with success the race of fulfilling God's purposes for our lives, and he contrasts our reward, which is imperishable, with the reward of an athlete, which is perishable. But don't miss what Paul said in the midst of his exhortation: athletes who compete in the games (similar to the Olympics today) exercise self-control in all things. So do we! As translated in the New International Version, "*They do it* to get a crown that will not last, *but we do it* to get a crown that will last forever" (1 Cor. 9:25, emphasis added).

Paul says that we live our lives like athletes, being disciplined in all things. The difference is that *they are self-controlled* with an earthly reward in view whereas *we are self-controlled* with a heavenly reward in view. But both of us, the athletes and the believers, are called to live disciplined lives. And as followers of Jesus, we are expected to follow Paul's example, who said, "No sloppy living for me! I'm staying alert and in top condition" (1 Cor. 9:27, THE MESSAGE).

Can we say the same thing about ourselves? Are we disciplined in all things? Have we subdued our bodies (see 1 Corinthians 9:27 in the New English Translation) when it comes to food? Do we practice self-denial when it comes to eating?

Proverbs gives us a strong warning about being out of control with our appetites when in the presence of rulers: "When you sit to eat with a ruler, consider diligently [or carefully] what is before you; and put a knife to your throat, if you are a man given to appetite" (Prov. 23:1–2, MEV). As *The Pulpit Commentary* explains, "'Stab thy gluttony,' Wordsworth. Restrain thyself by the strongest measures, convince thyself that thou art in the utmost peril, if thou art a glutton or wine-bibber."[6] In the words of Matthew Henry, "The sin we are here warned against is luxury and sensuality, and the indulgence of the appetite in eating and drinking, a sin that most easily besets us."[7]

Gluttony is never a good thing in the Word. It says, for example, "Be not among drunkards or among gluttonous eaters of meat, for the drunkard and the glutton will come to poverty, and slumber will clothe them with rags" (Prov. 23:20–21). And, "The one who keeps the law is a son with understanding, but a companion of gluttons shames his father" (Prov. 28:7).

This is serious business, and it is anything but an abstract, spiritual concept. Consider the findings of a 2002 report claiming the health risks of obesity are "worse than smoking, drinking, or poverty":

Two RAND [Corporation] researchers, health economist Roland Sturm and psychiatrist Kenneth Wells, examined the comparative effects of obesity, smoking, heavy drinking, and poverty on chronic health conditions and health expenditures. Their finding: obesity is the most serious problem. It is linked to a big increase in chronic health conditions and significantly higher health expenditures. And it affects more people than smoking, heavy drinking, or poverty....What were their conclusions? "The study reveals that obesity is linked to very high rates of chronic illnesses—higher than living in poverty, and much higher than smoking or drinking."[8]

But there's more. Obesity is much more widespread than smoking, drinking, or poverty: "Not only does obesity have more negative health consequences than smoking, drinking, or poverty, it also affects more people. Approximately 23 percent of Americans are obese. An additional 36 percent are overweight. By contrast, only 6 percent are heavy drinkers, 19 percent are daily smokers, and 14 percent live in poverty."[9]

These stats, however, are now outdated, since the percentages of overweight and obese Americans are even higher today. According to a major government survey, the National Health and Nutrition Examination Survey, completed in 2009–2010:

- More than 2 in 3 adults are considered to be overweight or obese.

- More than 1 in 3 adults are considered to be obese.

- More than 1 in 20 adults are considered to have extreme obesity.

- About one-third of children and adolescents ages 6 to 19 are considered to be overweight or obese.

- More than 1 in 6 children and adolescents ages 6 to 19 are considered to be obese.[10]

The report also states that "Overweight and obesity are risk factors for type 2 diabetes, heart disease, high blood pressure, and other health problems,"[11] which include the following:

- Nonalcoholic fatty liver disease (excess fat and inflammation in the liver of people who drink little or no alcohol)

- Osteoarthritis (a health problem causing pain, swelling, and stiffness in one or more joints)

- Some types of cancer: breast, colon, endometrial (related to the uterine lining), and kidney

- Stroke[12]

Fast forward to 2016, and a June 7 headline on CNBC .com states, "America's Obesity Epidemic Hits a New High." According to the article, "The U.S. obesity epidemic continues to worsen: The latest reports show that 40 percent of U.S. women are obese, and American teenagers are also continuing to put on weight.... Overall 38 percent of U.S. adults are obese and 17 percent of teenagers are, the two reports find.... Another third or so of Americans are overweight."[13] So, according to the most recent studies, roughly seven-in-ten Americans are either overweight or obese. This is staggering, even devastating, news.

If we just focus on the number of Americans who die of heart disease and then recognize the connection between unhealthy eating and heart disease, we will be sobered. As Dr. Fuhrman writes:

> Heart disease is the number one killer in the United States, accounting for more than 40 percent of all deaths. Each year approximately 1.5 million Americans suffer a heart attack or myocardial infarction (MI); nearly 500,000 of them die as a result. Most of these

deaths occur soon after the onset of symptoms and well before victims are admitted to a hospital. Every single one of those heart attacks is a terrible tragedy, as it could have been avoided.[14]

From Nancy: To reiterate what many medical professionals have said (and clinically proven), diseases such as diabetes, heart disease, and high blood pressure are primarily brought on by overweight, obesity, and unhealthy eating—and our overweight, obesity, and unhealthful eating are entirely under our control. We don't have to succumb to these illnesses if we choose rightly. It's entirely up to us. So, do we choose those things that do our bodies good or do we choose what does them harm? It's our choice alone.

As a lifelong chocoholic, I used to joke about the names of some of my favorite desserts: Death by Chocolate, Chocolate Decadence, Chocolate Suicide. I would ask, "Why do only the chocolate desserts have these names? Why not Tiramisu Suicide or Death by Apple Pie?" But this was no joking matter. These desserts were doing me no good, and they were far more death-giving than life-giving.

Many years ago I ran an errand for Nancy at the local grocery store, picking up some items we needed in the house. While shopping, I noticed a display with chocolate fudge (this is "hard core" stuff for a chocoholic) and decided I really needed a small chunk of it. The only problem was that this was supposed to be a "no sweets" time for me. Well, as I was checking out of the store, the cashier picked up the fudge and said to me, "Mmmm, good!" And then—to my shock—she looked at me and said, "Sinful!" Little did she know it, but she was right.

Again, I'm not here to play the Holy Spirit or to be your judge. And it would have been one thing if you or I indulged in eating unhealthy treats once or twice in a year. But for me, it was a daily habit, one that I was addicted to, and one that was doing me no good at all. What are the destructive eating habits in your own life?

ARE YOU A SLAVE TO YOUR APPETITE?

Headlines like these, which can easily be found everywhere online and which reflect thousands of articles and studies, offer a small sampling of the dangers of our typical diet:

- Just two [rations] of bacon a day raises your risk of cancer: Health chiefs put processed meat at same level as cigarettes.[15]

- Fat around the middle can "double the risk of early death."[16]

- The world now has a sweet tooth: Soaring sales of soft drinks and more sugar in foods is contributing to a "growing crisis in obesity, diabetes and heart disease."[17]

- Cancer ISN'T all in your genes: Up to 90 percent of cases "could be wiped out by avoiding triggers caused by our unhealthy lifestyles."[18]

- Revealed, your body on sugar: From weakening the immune system to triggering thrush, this terrifying tool reveals exactly how the white stuff harms our health.[19]

From Nancy: Again, all this is within our control. Do we choose those things that do our bodies good or choose what does them harm? It's our choice alone.

There are also the countless articles on health-promoting websites (such as DrFuhrman.com), with posts like, "The Standard American Diet Is Shortening Our Children's Lives." There Dr. Fuhrman writes that this current generation of children may not outlive their parents:

> The poor dietary habits of today's children [are] contributing to their obesity, chronic illness, and ill-health. [They are] also laying a foundation for poor academic performance, chronic disease later in life, violent behavior, and premature death. But children are not making these choices on their own; children's dietary habits are ingrained by their parents.[20]

If all this is true—and the scientific and anecdotal evidence is really impossible to deny—then we can't go on in willful ignorance, as I did for years. We must ask ourselves if the way we are eating is in harmony with our biblical calling, a calling that includes discipline and self-control. In fact, according to Paul, one of the fruits of the spirit is self-control (Gal. 5:23), with the Greek word meaning "restraint of one's emotions, impulses, or desires, *self-control*."[21] As one commentator explains, "'Self-control'...denotes control of more sensual passions than anger."[22]

When it comes to your eating habits, do you have self-control? When it comes to the passions of the flesh for unhealthy food, are you disciplined? Are you controlling your appetite or is your appetite controlling you? Some of us say that we're willing to die for Jesus, but we're not willing to control our appetites for Him (or, at the least, we're not willing to make a serious effort to control those appetites). This simply doesn't line up. We sing, "I surrender all," but we practice, "I surrender some." Or maybe we want to surrender but find ourselves helpless and bound.

Notice what Paul has to say about dangerous false teachers:

"For many are walking in such a way that they are the enemies of the cross of Christ. I have told you of them often and tell you again, even weeping. Their destination is destruction, their god is their appetite, their glory is in their shame, their minds are set on earthly things" (Phil 3:18–19, MEV). Or, as the relevant phrase is rendered in different versions: "their god is their stomach" (HCSB); they "make their bellies their gods" (THE MESSAGE); "whose God *is* the stomach" (LEB). How interesting that these heretics were also slaves to food!

Does that describe you? Is your stomach your god? Are you a slave to your appetite?

If so, I have good news for you: God is not condemning you! Instead, He is offering you a better way, a way of discipline, self-control, healthy eating, and vibrant life. But if He has convicted you through this chapter, I encourage you to confess your bad eating habits as sin, asking the Father for mercy and forgiveness, believing that Jesus paid for this sin as well, and trusting God for grace to overcome. With His help and with a good plan, you can do it!

So cast off the condemnation (when the Lord forgives, He really forgives), stop beating yourself up, and determine to quit making excuses for being overweight. There is a lot of light at the end of the tunnel, and every day you take a step in the right direction, that light will shine brighter and brighter. Forward!

From Nancy: For me, knowing God was not pleased with my eating habits was not enough to motivate or change me. I knew it was wrong, but I kept doing it. And knowing that He was tender and loving didn't change my behavior either. Whether God was pleased or displeased had no bearing on my behavior at all.

There are so many other areas in our lives, sad to say, that are just like this. We know it's wrong to gossip, but we just have to say that one little thing to our friend even when we know we shouldn't. And what about losing our temper or many other sins? We know they're wrong, but we do them anyway. We lack in prayer and reading the Word, and give priority to other things and feel guilty about it, but we continue on. The guilt doesn't seem to change us or our behavior, nor does His love and acceptance.

Knowing and understanding the things that displease the Lord did not seem to be a deterrent for me, so spiritual "remedies" were of little benefit. I had to do something in the natural that would help me to get a grip on my eating, and that, in turn, helped my spiritual life. I may be different than many, but for me, getting some practical help and guidance to get my eating under control was the thing that positively fueled my spiritual life. When my eating was out of control, everything was out of control. The house wasn't as clean, work piled up, tasks were left undone—my entire life became undisciplined and unbalanced. But when the eating was under control, everything changed and my life ran like a well-oiled machine. When my eating was not right, nothing went right, and when my eating was corrected, everything else righted itself.

That's just the way it worked in my life. All the preaching and teaching and spiritualizing the problem did not help me. I needed practical, commonsense tips and tools to help me gain control. And when I learned those tips, God was there to strengthen me and help me use them. But He was the One who taught me what to do. When I sought Him in prayer, He showed me His plan for maintaining a healthy lifestyle, customized just for me.

QUESTIONS FOR REFLECTION

1. What Scripture verse spoke to you most strongly in this chapter?

2. Do you recognize unhealthy eating to be sinful just as watching pornography, gossiping about your neighbor, cheating on your spouse, or getting drunk are all sinful?

3. Have you received forgiveness from the Lord for unhealthy eating? Jesus died for this sin too! Have you forgiven yourself for it?

4. Do you believe the lie that your stomach is your god, or are you renewing your mind with God's Word, having died to sin with Jesus, and now living in newness of life with Him?

CHAPTER 4

CHANGING YOUR
MIND ABOUT FOOD

BEFORE I GET back to my own story, let me share
with you some important spiritual principles when it
comes to food since, oddly enough, we often don't
think about food in spiritual terms. We eat several times a
day, food plays a major role in our lives, and it is often a central part of our church gatherings and fellowships, yet we
tend to think of food in nonspiritual terms. In the same way,
we often think of the consequences of our bad food choices—
our fat—in nonspiritual terms. That's why many of us just
accept our obesity and our food addictions as being part of
who we are. This is a big mistake.

For example, we think of certain people as fat and others as
thin, as if this was no different than them being tall or short,
but the two categories are quite different. In the vast majority
of cases, being fat or thin is due to choices we make; being
tall or short has nothing to do with our choices. That's just
the way God made us, but He didn't make us fat, nor does
He want us to be fat. Well-fed (in terms of having enough
good food to eat to sustain maximum health), yes; fat, no.

I'm fully aware that some people are thin because of their metabolism, and they can eat lots of food—even unhealthy food—and remain thin. But that's no excuse for those of us with slower metabolisms to eat the way they eat, nor is it a matter of being "fair." Life is not fair, and more importantly, God's grace is more than enough to level things out. And the reality is, as we get older, we can't get away with eating the way we did when we were young. In fact, the reality is that we never get away with eating poorly, even those who have a fast metabolism. Bad eating habits will ultimately take their toll, resulting in all kinds of preventable diseases.

I used to think to myself, "Well, I don't eat certain foods. That's just the way I am. I have limited tastes"—as if that's the way God created my taste buds. I thought some people, like my father and sister, eat just about anything while other people, like my mom and me, are very picky eaters. That's just the way we are, and that's how we live our lives. It's not right or wrong or good or bad. It just is, and there's no way to change it.

Says who? Where in the Word—or in science—is that written? Where it is written that tastes can't be changed, that the palate can't be retrained? I've been studying the Scriptures for forty years now, and nowhere does it say, "You can change your interests and your desires by renewing your mind according to the Word, you can break sinful habits, you can go from being carnal to spiritual, but you can never change your eating habits or your tastes." Nowhere is that written, not in the Bible and not in our biology. We can change our eating habits, our food tastes, and our relationship to food as a whole, and get this—we can do it in our own human strength, just as we can do physical exercises in our human strength (unless we have a physical handicap).

We can choose to take a walk. We can choose to start jogging (again, unless we have a physical limitation). We can choose to go to the gym and work out. And we can choose to eat differently. Why do we put food into a different category?

When we first start exercising, our body doesn't want to respond. But as we persevere, our body falls into line. It's the same with eating. With perseverance, our habits can dramatically change.

You say, "Dr. Brown, you don't understand. I'm totally bound here. I've tried to make changes a hundred times over, and I actually gag on some healthy foods. Trust me on this. If I could change, I would. I hate being fat."

Honestly, I understand what you are saying! I did gag trying brussels sprouts years ago. I did pray that God would help me to love broccoli the way I loved chocolate, and I saw no change in my desires whatsoever. And I was addicted to certain foods, and I hated being fat. I do understand.

But that's the whole purpose of this chapter (and, really, this whole book). I want to encourage you to think about your food habits, addictions, and weaknesses in spiritual terms. The same way you overcome other sins and develop new, wholesome habits is the same way you change your relationship to food. So let's start changing our minds about food together. For the remainder of this chapter, I am going to highlight eight truths that you must realize (and accept!) in order to change the way you think about food.

JESUS DIED FOR THE SIN OF OVEREATING

First, if overeating and/or unhealthy eating is a sin, did Jesus die for that sin? Did He pay for it in full on the cross? When you confess it to Him as sin and ask for forgiveness, does He wash you clean and forgive you, even if you keep messing up and seeking His mercy? The answer is yes, yes, and yes. He forgives the sin of overeating just like He forgives the sin of pornography or the sin of lying.

Perhaps by putting food into a different category you fail to receive forgiveness from the Father, and your fat is a constant reminder to you that you're an unclean sinner, whereas if you lie to someone then confess that sin to them and to God, you can walk away feeling forgiven. But you wear your fat 24/7.

So start by renewing your mind and confessing your eating sins to the Lord, receiving mercy and grace from heaven. "For we do not have a high priest who is unable to sympathize with our weaknesses, but one who in every respect has been tempted as we are, yet without sin. Let us then with confidence draw near to the throne of grace, that we may receive mercy and find grace to help in time of need" (Heb. 4:15–16).

YOUR FAT DOES NOT DEFINE YOU

Second, your fat does not define you. I'm aware it's with you all the time, not just in appearance but in tangible feeling. (Nancy articulates this clearly in her story; her fat physically bothered her every moment of the day, restricting her movements and her freedom and even her being comfortable.) But being overweight doesn't define you. Being a child of God defines you. Being a new creation in Jesus defines you. Being in Him—seated with Him in heavenly places—defines you. So rather than thinking about yourself as a fat person—in a way that defines, describes, and delineates you—think of yourself as a beloved child of the Father who has a weight issue to deal with.

I'm not talking about denying reality. I'm not talking about rebuking calories before you eat (yes, some believers actually do this!) or of confessing, "I'm thin in the Spirit" (I know someone who did this too; the fact is that your spirit is not operating in the realm of physical weight). I'm talking about not allowing a negative, destructive, hopeless, harmful self-image to dominate your psyche so that your overweight defines the essence of who you are. Instead, let your standing with God fundamentally define you. Then from that point of confidence in the Lord, you can address the very real problem of being overweight.

YOU ARE AN OVERCOMER IN CHRIST

Third, in Jesus you are an overcomer. In Jesus, you are dead to sin. In Jesus, you are not a slave to the passions and lusts of the flesh. As Paul wrote to the Galatians, "And those who belong to Christ Jesus have crucified the flesh with its passions and desires" (Gal. 5:24). That includes you and me, and you need to think in terms of having victory over food just as you have victory over drugs or alcohol or gambling or porn. Tell that food, "You are not my master." Look in the mirror and say, "My stomach is not my god." Walk around your house worshipping and praising God, saying, "In Jesus, I can be free from food addictions! In Jesus, I am not a slave! God's grace is more than enough!"

From Nancy: My fat didn't define me in terms of it being who I was. Being obese felt very foreign to me, like I was in someone else's body. This was not how my life was supposed to be—it was an aberration, and that's what made it such an overpoweringly negative thing; it wasn't me! Every day I spent in that body was disorienting, like being in the wrong place. So this is a different side of the same coin. Some people view themselves as overweight and think they'll always be that way—it's just who they are. I never viewed myself like that. I always expected that I would be thin and would not go to my grave a fat lady.

GRACE EMPOWERS YOU TO LIVE ABOVE SIN

Fourth, recognize that the grace that saved you from sin is the same grace that empowers you to live above sin, including the sin of unhealthy eating. Recognize that everything you need to overcome food addictions and to be free and to renew your mind and to change your palate is found in the Lord.

The Spirit living inside of you is more than enough to carry you to victory. I am a living witness!

As Paul wrote to Titus, "For the grace of God has appeared, bringing salvation for all people, training us to renounce ungodliness and worldly passions, and to live *self-controlled*, upright, and godly lives in the present age, waiting for our blessed hope, the appearing of the glory of our great God and Savior Jesus Christ, who gave himself for us to redeem us from all lawlessness and to purify for himself a people for his own possession who are zealous for good works" (Titus 2:11–14, emphasis added).

Or, in the words of Peter, "His divine power has granted to us *all things that pertain to life and godliness*, through the knowledge of him who called us to his own glory and excellence, by which he has granted to us his precious and very great promises, so that through them you may become partakers of the divine nature, having escaped from the corruption that is in the world because of sinful desire" (2 Pet. 1:3–4, emphasis added). When he speaks of "all things that pertain to life and godliness," he is including the very real issue of bad eating habits. And when he speaks of "precious and very great promises," he is including promises that help us change our relationship to food.

From Nancy: When you think that God, the Creator of the heavens and the earth, has made a way for His divine nature to live in us, could that nature ever eat the way I did? Impossible. That is not God's divine nature. When we get a real glimpse of the beauty of His nature, we come to realize that a lot of what we do is very foreign to it. It is certainly not God's nature living through us that is stuffing and gorging ourselves. It's our ugly flesh. We do need to learn how to let God dominate us so that He shines through. But understanding how to live with God's essence living in and through us and emanating out of us is much more than we can tackle in this book.

FREEDOM THROUGH OBEDIENCE IS A CHOICE

Fifth, if you realize that unhealthy eating is a sin (as emphasized in the last chapter), then this is not just a matter of victory and freedom. It's a matter of obedience. Will you obey your Lord when it comes to eating? Will you say no to the flesh and yes to your Savior? Perhaps you need some spiritual backbone here. Perhaps rather than just excusing this as a weakness, you need to deal with this as a serious spiritual matter. I often hear obese believers (including pastors) joke about their bad food choices as if it's nothing, saying, "I love my ice cream!" Would they say just as freely, "I love my porn!"? I think not!

From Nancy: Would these believers and pastors say, "I love my ice cream!" from their hospital beds after their chests have been cracked open as a result of coronary bypass surgery? Would they be so flippant? They are flippant about it because they don't take seriously the negative consequences of decades of ice cream indulgence (along with all the other poor dietary choices they have made through the years). And they don't really believe it will happen to them. It sounds silly to be so serious about ice cream, and it's easy to joke about it while sitting comfortably at the dinner table. But it all looks entirely different when someone is suffering the consequences of those choices. Unfortunately, many people suffer, and tragedy strikes before they wake up and take things seriously. I write this not to condemn, as I likely could have eaten many of them under the table in my former days! I fully understand how foreign the thought of giving up a food can be.

You might ask, "When does eating become a sin? Obviously we all need to eat, and it's hard to imagine we can eat perfectly healthy foods in the perfect proportions all the time. So how do we gauge what's sinful?"

Without trying to play the Holy Spirit in your life, I would suggest these guidelines:

1. If the way you're eating (or, specifically, what you're eating) is causing you to be seriously overweight or, worse still, making you physically ill, could it be sinful?

2. If you're eating foods the Lord has convicted you not to eat, could it be sinful?

3. If you're being a glutton, gorging yourself until you're totally stuffed, could it be sinful?

4. If you're eating foods to satisfy an unhealthy addiction, could it be sinful?

5. If you're eating in secret and hiding food, could it be sinful?

SPIRITUAL WARFARE REGARDING FOOD IS REAL

Sixth, recognize the reality of spiritual warfare when it comes to food. I don't want to overly spiritualize things here, but I don't want to leave out very real spiritual truths. Of course Satan tempts us with food. Of course our bondage is both physical and spiritual. Of course we can break these strongholds in Jesus's name through prayer, leading to a changed lifestyle. Prayer alone won't do the trick; it takes prayer and obedience. Why not attack demonic food strongholds the way you would attack a satanic stronghold that was trying to destroy one of your kids? It's the same devil we're dealing with and the same Jesus who triumphs over that devil. And we triumph in Him. (To read the steps Nancy took to recognize the stronghold of food in her life and break its power, see appendix B.)

WITH GOD ALL THINGS ARE POSSIBLE!

Seventh, believe that with God all things are possible! This is a fundamental truth of the Word of God and is as surely true as God is God. (See Jeremiah 32, Matthew 17, Mark 9, and Luke 1.) Nothing is impossible with the Lord—including you changing your relationship to food, including you being free from food addictions, including you loving healthy foods, including you being thin and fit and energized. It's possible!

[handwritten margin note: Including me adoring my husband!]

I have as many excuses as anyone (see chapter 13)—traveling constantly, having grown up eating a very limited diet, being addicted to chocolate and sweets for decades, and having had overall bad eating habits for the first fifty-nine years of my life. Do you know how wonderful it is to desire apples the way I used to desire sweets? Do you know how good it feels to sit in a restaurant and enjoy a healthy salad while others sit at the table with me eating unhealthy foods, telling me that they know they need to change and asking me how I have so much energy and seem so alive?

One of my closest friends traveled the world with me serving as my personal assistant, and he knows well what my eating habits were. And Nancy, my bride of more than forty years, completely gave up on trying to get me to eat new foods, knowing what a baby I was when it came to this. (And hey, I used to think, "That's the way God made my palate, right? I just don't like certain foods!") How different my life has become, and how wonderful are the benefits.

I remember going into a grocery store to get some salad items while on the road one time. As I picked out the lettuce and spinach and cucumbers and onions and tomatoes and red and green and yellow peppers and other items, I said to myself, "We are going to have a feast!" I was genuinely excited about it.

In the past, I would have been looking for the nearest pizzeria or, if I had more time, getting myself some massive chicken parmesan meal, but only after loading up on bread and butter (of course, with a small salad too), then getting some luscious, decadent chocolate dessert and some unhealthy snacks for my room. Now, I'm munching on blueberries and looking for a place that can make me a healthy smoothie, and I'm enjoying what I eat. All things are possible! (Nancy tells me this is truly a miracle!)

From Nancy: I have to be honest here. The bad foods still look and smell really, really good to me. I still wish I could eat them. That's probably not what you wanted to hear. You most likely wanted me to say that I have no interest in bad foods, that I have no temptations, and that it's always easy. It's not so easy. It takes a lot of determination and hard work, but most of the things in life that produce the greatest fruit require the greatest effort. But the reward is all the more exquisite!

Yes, I thoroughly enjoy the healthy foods, but there is still that pull toward the unhealthy ones. Most former addicts, such as alcoholics, can still be attracted to what used to addict them. There is still that lure, that pull, so they have to protect themselves. It's not a sin to be tempted. The fleshly pull can still be there, which is why it is so important to use wisdom and common sense to help keep yourself from falling into temptation. There have been times when I have refused a dinner invitation because I knew I was feeling vulnerable and my flesh was craving the wrong things. I can't help the cravings. I can't wish them away, and I don't feel guilty for them either. They just come sometimes. But I use the wisdom God gave me to protect myself in a weak moment. Know your weaknesses and protect yourself. Thankfully, over time, the temptations get less and less frequent, but that doesn't mean they entirely disappear (although for some, they do).

✝ HEALTHY EATING IS ✘ COOPERATING WITH THE LORD

Eighth, look at healthy eating as cooperating with the Lord, as working with Him for your good and the good of those you love. There are some meals I enjoy more than others, but I especially thank God for the super-healthy meals that I don't enjoy quite as much as the others, particularly some soups that Nancy makes for me. I was never much of a soup eater (other than wonton soup at a Chinese restaurant), and somehow the look of these mega-healthy soups didn't appeal to me so much at first.

So when I would sit down to eat one of these meals, I would say, "Father, thank You so much for this amazing, healthy soup. Thank You for the incredible nourishment that is in this meal and that will help me run my race. I know it gives me an advantage when I work out; I know it helps me when I travel overseas; I know it enhances me when I sit down to write. Thank You, Lord, for this food!" And it is food for which we can be thankful. (By the way, those soups have become more and more appealing to me over time.)

It's time to change your mind about food and to approach it from a spiritual point of view. You'll be blessed as you do.

From Nancy: When it comes to changing our relationship to food, we must realize that food is not the center of our lives. It is not the end-all. So much of our lives revolve around eating and tasting and pleasing our palates. We mainly eat for pleasure, not for health or true nourishment. Most of our eating is because we want something tasty, not because we're truly hungry. Personally, I was never hungry because I never went long enough without food to be seriously hungry. Eating always had to be a taste sensation. It's nice to be in a place where food is not the all-consuming, central theme. You enjoy your meals, but food is put in its proper, divinely ordained place. It's a very freeing place.

QUESTIONS FOR REFLECTION

1. Which of the eight points listed in this chapter spoke to you the most strongly? Why do you think that was?

2. Have you looked at your food issues through entirely natural eyes? Can you see how important it is to see things through spiritual eyes?

3. Does your fat define you? Can you see how changing your sense of identity can liberate you?

4. Do you really believe you can make a radical change with God's help? If not, talk to Him honestly about it and meditate on the life-changing power of His grace.

CHAPTER 5

TOO FAT TO FLY

T HE WORDS WERE spoken clearly, carefully, and with great conviction: "Brethren, we are too fat to fly."

It was a Sunday night late in 1982, and we had gathered to pray together for a few hours in the midst of a wonderful spiritual visitation that our congregation was experiencing. These Sunday night prayer meetings had become the highlight of the week as we would come together in great anticipation, not knowing what would happen as we prayed.

Lost sinners came to faith during the prayer meeting. Sick bodies were healed. Believers came to deep repentance and were mightily filled with the Spirit.

But on this particular night, something was missing. The meeting was flat, lacking vitality, and there was a heaviness in the air. That's when one of the men there spoke these words: "Brethren, we are too fat to fly. We've had our nice, big meals today before coming here, and now we're so full of food that we're tired and lethargic."

Put another way, you can't walk in the Spirit if you indulge the flesh, and that's exactly what we had done that night. Like an overgorged bird, we were too fat to fly.

A few years later I received an invitation to speak at a luncheon event for a women's ministry, and I asked one of my students to come along for the meeting. As we drove together, the Lord laid a message on my heart with the title, "Too Fat to Fly." (Remember that I was on my way to speak at a luncheon, presumably at a nice restaurant too.) When I told the student what I was going to preach on, he asked me lightheartedly if I wanted to reconsider the title, and we smiled at the thought, knowing how inappropriate it might sound.

Interestingly, the message was not related to food—I was talking about the spiritual principle of being so weighed down with the things of the world that we were too fat to "fly" in God. But I became very uncomfortable when I met the pastor who was overseeing the meeting: he was a very overweight brother with a great big smile.

When it came time to have lunch (which took place before the message), this pastor was asked to give thanks, and he began by saying, "Lord, You know how much I love food!" And I was about to get up and preach on being too fat to fly!

Well, I still used that title and preached on that theme, being very careful to say I was *not* talking about food—I really didn't want to embarrass this brother, and in those days I was fairly thin myself, despite my unhealthy eating habits. But now I *do* want to focus on food since overeating (or eating to satisfy our lusts rather than enhance our health) is a real detriment to our spiritual lives.

I absolutely believe that God has given us richly all things to enjoy (1 Tim. 6:17), and I don't accept the idea that it is sinful to enjoy food (or other things in this world). I don't believe we need to go around sulking and mourning all the time, as if it's wrong to experience any natural pleasure.

But I do believe it's wrong to cater to the flesh, to feed our lusts, to be enslaved by habits, to have food addictions, and to live an indulgent life—by which I mean a life that is lacking in self-denial, a life in which we live to eat rather than eat to live, a life that is clearly not ruled by the Spirit when it comes to diet. Do you concur?

When our daughters were little, we were driving one night as a family to a midweek church service where I was going to preach when we stopped along the way to get some ice cream. We had a pretty long drive to the meeting—almost an hour—and then it would be another hour into the service before I would preach, but that was not enough time for me to digest fully that chocolate ice cream cone. It sat there in my stomach as I preached, and I did not feel as free as I normally did, nor did I feel as in tune with the Spirit as I was used to feeling. The flesh got in the way!

All of us have experienced something like that in our lives, even if we've never preached. We have a giant lunch, stuffing ourselves with our favorite delicacies, only to feel terribly sluggish through the afternoon. We enjoy a few days of feasting around the holidays, only to feel miserable afterward (leading, of course, to our next failed attempt to diet to shed the extra weight).

What I'm suggesting is that, in many ways, we live *our entire lives* like that—feeling weighed down and sluggish—yet some of us are so used to it that we're not even aware of it. Or we're aware of that constant feeling of being tired and run-down, but we don't know what's causing it. So we try new meds or vitamins, or we have a long talk with the doctor, or we concentrate on getting more sleep.

Of course, there could be other reasons for our sluggishness—we could be sick or sleep-deprived. But all things being equal, indulging the flesh will ground us; eating in a disciplined, healthy way will give us wings. Wouldn't it be great to fly again, to have a youthful vigor you haven't known in years? Wouldn't it be great to have a sharper mind, an energized attitude, and a renewed zest for life?

From Nancy: It's hard to explain how incredible it feels to get rid of that heavy load. It changes everything. I used to wake up every day not believing that this thin body was actually mine. Every morning I was surprised to be thin, since it was such a foreign thing. But oh, how wonderful it felt—and it feels!

LET GOD GIVE YOU WINGS

A few years back, I developed a little exercise routine to use on the road, giving me a full-body workout that I could do in my hotel room. It consists of jumping jacks (two count as one), air squats (where you crouch down as if about to sit in a chair and then stand up), pushups, and stomach crunches (lying on your back and touching your knees to your elbows, with your hands clasped behind your head). You start with twenty reps of each exercise (meaning forty jumping jacks and twenty of the other three), then nineteen of each, then eighteen, then seventeen, counting all the way down until you reach one (which means at the end, you're constantly up and down).

I had done this for a couple of years while heavy, shooting for a time a little over twenty minutes, during which I would do a total of 420 jumping jacks and 210 of each of the other three exercises—quite a strenuous routine, with no breaks taken other than to breathe deeply a few times along the way. After losing a lot of weight (I was not at my goal yet, but I had lost a lot already), I decided to do the exercise routine in my hotel while on the road ministering, and I couldn't believe how I felt. I was flying!

Of course, I had to push hard to finish strong, and it took a certain amount of discipline, but, overall, it was surprisingly easy, and the difference in how I felt was absolutely dramatic. It was wonderful! And that's a picture of how life feels in general for me: the difference is absolutely dramatic. (For those who are competitive, my best time now is 12:58, so have at it. And don't worry about your form; just keep moving.)

To illustrate the point about the extra weight we carry, I encourage you to determine how much overweight you are (for guidelines, see appendix C) then to go to a gym where there are free weights (in other words, dumbbells and the like), and if you're able, pick up that amount of weight. In other words, if you're 50 pounds overweight, pick up a twenty-five-pound dumbbell in each hand. Then walk around for a little while. Or if there are steps nearby (again, *only* if you're healthy enough to do this without a problem), go up and down the steps, or do some squats holding the weight in your hands.

On the one hand, this will give you an exaggerated feeling, since spreading the weight over your entire body will not feel as severe as carrying it in a concentrated way with dumbbells (plus this is actually adding to your current weight). On the other hand, it's the same additional weight, and we are stressing our heart and our blood vessels and other parts of our body (such as our back and knees) by carrying this unnecessary and, frankly, very unhealthy baggage. We are just too fat to fly—or, at the least, to fly as high and freely and successfully as God intends us to. Is it worth losing parts of your spiritual destiny and calling for the sake of food?

When I had lost fifty pounds, I asked my family to take a twenty-five-pound dumbbell in each hand and walk around. They were shocked at the amount of weight, as was I. When I had lost sixty pounds, I asked our grandson Andrew to get on my back (he weighed about sixty pounds at the time), and I did pushups with him on my back. Not easy! Then, with him clinging to my back, I walked up and down the stairs. How in the world did I live like that for years?

When I had lost more than ninety pounds, I asked who in the family could pick up forty-five-pound dumbbells with each hand (not many takers, except for my son-in-law Ryan, who wanted to be sure I mentioned him in this book). Yet *this* (and more) was what I was carrying around on my frame for many, many months, all while working out and keeping up a nonstop ministry schedule, and all while getting more and more tired, having less and less energy, becoming somewhat weary of life, and, more dangerously still, having my blood pressure rising steadily.

Now I have wings to fly and soar and glide, and I'm thriving more than I can remember in many years—all because of a radical change in my relationship to food. The same can happen to you!

There's no reason to be too fat to fly. The Lord wants to give you some wings—and I don't mean buffalo wings!

Even professional athletes can get too fat to fly. As Charles Barkley of NBA fame commented, "You can't make a living playing basketball if you are fat or out of shape."[1] As for the players who were overweight and still successful, another retired NBA star explained, "They could be somewhat effective, but they were never as good as they could be. And, eventually, it catches up with you."[2] And what have these players concluded now that they are retired from the NBA? "The older they get, the more diligently they have to watch their diet."[3]

As this book unfolds, I'll explain in greater detail how my life changed so dramatically, but first, I want to let you in on something I've never shared publicly before, at least in any kind of detail. In short, if there was a shortcut to health, I tried it. And the results were never what I hoped. Keep reading to find out more!

QUESTIONS FOR REFLECTION

1. How has unhealthy eating negatively affected your spiritual life? In what ways has it made you too fat to fly?

2. How has unhealthy eating negatively affected your social life?

3. If someone paid you one million dollars to reach your ideal weight and then paid you that same amount every year to maintain it, do you think you would do it? If so, isn't your health and your freedom and your obedience to God more important than one million dollars?

4. Imagine yourself thin and vibrant. What are the first things you would do in your new body? If you can't imagine yourself thin and vibrant, ask the Lord for help you get to the root of this negativity and then ask Him to help you get that positive, healthy picture in your mind. He didn't make you to be fat!

CHAPTER 6

ANTI-FAT CREAM AND THE MAGIC ENERGY PILL

FOR MOST OF my adult life I looked for something to boost my energy, not because I was lethargic but because I live such a full life and push myself very hard. If only I could get an energy boost!

I wasn't looking for a new high, as if I wanted to find a legal substitute for methamphetamines (especially methedrine), which I used to shoot or snort as a teenager before I knew the Lord. No, I just wanted some healthy energy, and I tried just about everything I could get my hands on, including the latest vitamin supplement, energy drink, or the like.

When it came to losing weight, I also looked for a cheap and easy fix. One pill promised to boost your metabolism while you slept. Wonderful! I could eat what I wanted during the day and take this pill before bedtime and, voila, I'd be thin almost overnight. Another pill promised to provide all the fruits and vegetables I needed in one day. Perfect! I could not imagine eating so many fruits and vegetables in a week (or even a month), let alone do it every day. This pill would do the trick!

One time while flying, I was flipping through the airline magazine when I discovered the most amazing thing yet. (This is really embarrassing, but I'm going to tell the story anyway.) It was a special cream that you would apply to the fat parts of your body, and if you did it regularly, the fat would be reduced. I kid you not! (From Nancy: I can't believe I'm reading this!)

Well, the embarrassing thing is not that I read about this product but that I actually bought it, without telling Nancy. (How in the world could I tell her I did something so stupid?) Unfortunately, using this cream was quite uncomfortable, since there was never a really good time to put it on, day or night. It was greasy and would stick to your clothes, pajamas, or bed sheets, and since the whole key was to apply it and leave it on, you were stuck for hours with this gooey cream on your legs or stomach or wherever you applied it. I don't think I even tried it more than a couple of times before realizing how idiotic this was, telling Nancy about it, and then throwing it way. What a joke!

Unfortunately I wasn't the only one looking for a quick fix. As summer drew near in 2015, I began to track e-mails that came into my junk folder promising rapid solutions to body fat along with painless solutions to diabetes and heart disease. Here's a sampling from one day within a seventy-five minute time span:

Sage-Hull
Mayo Clinic Document-Get Rid of Diabetes within 2.5 weeks   12:40 PM
A Scientific Mayo Document Specifies How to Get Rid of from All Forms of

---

OmegaK
Discover the FREE Trick For Preventing Heart Attacks #1234079   12:34PM
Can this 10 Second Trick Help Prevent YOUR Heart Attack?

Slimmer by Summer
Burn Your Jelly-Belly with No Special Food or Exercise, Coupon expires 04.28   12:27 PM
Do This Once a Day to be Slim by Summer. Coupon ends 04.28.2015

Diminish Wrinkles
New Way to Safely Remove Unsightly Wrinkles, Risk-free Trial expires Today   12:20 PM
Look 20 Years younger in minutes! Risk-free Sample ends 28Apr2015

Drops Waist Size
Consumer Results: "I shed 6 lbs int he first 15 days" - Free Sample   11:44 AM
"I shed 6 lbs in the first 15 days."

Eat Carbs Drop lbs
GNC's new carb controller will melt 22lbs/month - 6518930   11:40 AM
The Doctor's review new carb filter - proven to drop 4lbs/week. GO HERE

Flat Bikini Belly
Feeling flabby? Drop 14# of bellyflab in 14 days. Free Trial Today Only #1069   11:34 AM
Start your Free Trial by 28April2015 and Drop 22# by Summer

One exercise ad promised this: "60-second morning routine KILLS, High Blood Pressure & Reverses 20 Years of Deadly Belly Fat." All that in just one minute per day! Other e-mails featured special "tricks" and "secrets"—all yours for just a few bucks. And the same seductive message is always there—this time, one of these will work for you, even though none of the other gimmicks worked before, all while you're bypassing the one thing that will work: radically changing your lifestyle!

Returning back to my own story, and thinking back to the time I bought that anti-fat cream, you need to realize that virtually no one thought of me at that time (somewhere around 2000) as being obese. I may have been forty to fifty pounds overweight, but standing almost 6'3," I certainly didn't look terrible. Yet, as I shared earlier, I hated being fat and was bothered by it all the time, hence the constant search for quick-fix remedies. Anything but radically changing my diet. In fact, about a decade later I gladly worked out several times a week for an hour at a time until I was ready to collapse rather than change my diet and lifestyle. In my mind, the workouts would take care of the weight loss; dietary change was just too difficult. (Obviously, I was wrong.)

And so, I tried lots of other gimmicks over the years. When my cholesterol and blood pressure started to get elevated, I took nonmedical supplements that were supposed to help adjust those levels. I didn't want to take prescription medication because of the many negative side effects, so I tried several different ones for years without the slightest evidence that they did any good.

One of my friends who had lost a lot of weight following a special program encouraged me to spend several hundred dollars and enroll myself in the program. The plan called on me to drink one of their "healthy" shakes in the morning (chocolate, of course). I could then eat what I wanted for lunch (within limits), not having to give up any of the foods I liked. Then I would drink one of the shakes at night. And best of all, they had some *delicious* and (supposedly) healthy chocolates that I could have (just not more than a couple per day; the portions were small). The problem was that the shakes were very expensive, I had some problems keeping up with the program on the road, and I saw very little change.

Although I'm pretty sure I would have lost some weight had I stayed on the program for a period of months, the facts are: 1) the shakes were nowhere as healthy as fruits, vegetables, and other healthy foods; 2) I was still eating unhealthy stuff that would ultimately clog my arteries and cause other problems; and 3) I would never have lost the full amount I needed to lose to get anywhere near my ideal weight.

From Nancy: There's no way you can stuff into a box, pill, or powder all the enzymes and phytochemicals contained in the plant foods we should be eating. They keep discovering new compounds every year and who knows how many are yet to be discovered. We cannot depend on a pill to provide all the necessary nutrients our body needs, hoping it will take up the slack for a nutrient-depleted diet. And downing a few tablets is not going to undo all the accumulated damage from decades of dietary abuse.

Over the years, I bought some diet books, looking for a new-fangled discovery that would allow me to eat what I wanted—with some minor changes along the way—and yet lose weight. One e-book I downloaded claimed to have the secret to weight loss, encouraging you to eat whatever you wanted with the exception that you change your schedule radically each day. This was supposed to get your metabolism to speed up. Wrong again! Another book told me that if I ate certain foods—including foods that I hated or had never tasted and never planned to taste—along with the foods I did like, the weight would come off. I didn't even bother trying that one.

One night in a hotel after speaking, I was unwinding before going to sleep and started watching an infomercial about the latest ab-reducing gadget. (It was that stomach fat that I hated and that embarrassed me.) I forget exactly what the product was, but if I used it to exercise every day, within weeks my stomach would be a few inches thinner, guaranteed. I fell asleep shortly after turning the commercial off, but when I woke up in the morning, I was very excited. I was about to be thin! I would be taking inches off my stomach! It was going to happen!

From Nancy: And this man has a PhD in ancient Semitic languages! It never ceased to amaze me not only that he would sneak all these crazy "miracle" products into our home, but also that he was actually gullible enough to fall for the sales pitch. I told him repeatedly they would never work, and, of course, they never did. The wife is always right, even without a PhD.

Apparently this persuasive infomercial got into my brain before I turned in, and when I woke up in the morning, I was totally sold. The brainwashing worked! When I realized what had happened, I was amazed at the power of advertising (and a little ashamed at my gullibility too). For the record, I didn't buy the gadget, whatever it was. (Also for the record, I virtually never watch infomercials. This time was an exception.)

I mentioned previously that, when working out, my trainer would say to me (and the other guys working out), "Abs are made in the kitchen." But surely, I thought, with some minor changes, like avoiding the really bad foods and cutting back on my overall caloric intake, my workouts would take care of my abs. Once again, I was wrong, although under the fat I had some pretty strong abdominal muscles. You just couldn't see them because of the extra, health-destroying fatty layers that covered them.

Of course, there were many times that I did make serious changes to my diet: no sweets for extended periods of time, "healthy" Subway sandwiches rather than pizza, reducing my caloric intake by one-third. The problem was that I would lose some weight—as much as thirty to forty pounds on a couple of occasions—but it would stop there and I would get discouraged, thinking, "I would just about have to starve myself to get down to my desired weight."

Actually, what I needed to do was stop eating the bad food and start eating the good food, things like raw nuts, which I couldn't just eat by the cupful. Once I made this radical change—out with the old and in with the new—the weight came off quickly and painlessly: ninety-five pounds in less than eight months. And it has stayed off painlessly as well. Best of all, I get to eat *lots* of healthy food every day, since the body is satisfied with bulk, not calories, meaning that I can have a giant smoothie in the morning, one that fills me up for a good five hours, and my caloric intake is less than 500 calories. Or I can have a delicious, *giant* salad for dinner (with a healthy, homemade dressing), filling a four-quart bowl and taking me about thirty minutes to eat, and yet it contains less than 400 calories—in other words, less than two small candy bars or two small bags of M&Ms. Which do you think will fill up your stomach more?

AN ABOUT-FACE

There's a spiritual principle to making such radical changes as well. If you're committing fornication and you want to get right with God, do you cut back on how many times you fornicate or do you ask the Lord for help and then stop sleeping around? It's the same with getting high or getting drunk or any other sinful practice. Does repentance mean doing it less or does it mean making an about-face and saying good-bye to the destructive habit? By God's grace, it means making a radical change and turning away from willful disobedience, not just reducing the amount of times we disobey the Lord.

But there's more. Do we just stiffen our resolve and say, "I won't do this anymore," or do we fill ourselves with the good things of God? Do we just say, "I'm done with getting drunk," or do we worship and commune with the Lord, read the Word and pray, walk in the fullness of the Spirit, and behold the beauty of Jesus? As Paul wrote to the Ephesians, "And do not get drunk with wine, for that is debauchery, but be filled with the Spirit" (Eph. 5:18). We stop doing what is bad by doing what is good. By turning away from what is wrong, we turn toward what is right.

It's the exact same thing with food. If you realize what you're eating is wrong or the amount you're eating is wrong, you will find freedom by making a complete about-face, replacing what is unhealthy with what is healthy, and before you know it, you'll be living a new life. Something happens when you make a radical break with the flesh. God will help you do it!

On and off over the years, I prayed that God would help me to love broccoli as much as I loved chocolate, but not once did my desire for chocolate lessen or my desire for broccoli increase. But when I quit eating chocolate and started feasting on salads (which included broccoli or broccoli sprouts), my desire for greens increased dramatically, and the satisfaction I have in eating them increased dramatically. Just as in the Bible, healings often came when people obeyed Christ's commands—"Stretch out your hand" or "Stand to your feet"—so also natural breakthroughs often come when we take that first step of obedience by faith.

From Nancy: You might think this is a hard pill to swallow. After all, what's wrong with having one tiny brownie or a piece of cake every now and then? They're not sinful. Having a small treat on a special occasion is not the problem. The problem is that many of us are unable to limit ourselves to that one occasion. It whets our appetite for more, and we find ourselves overeating or bingeing and being drawn into behaviors that are destructive. That's how it works with me. The highly palatable, salty, sugary, fat-laden foods have pulled me out of peaceful, controlled eating every single time I've eaten them in the last forty years. So why would I play with fire? Why would I eat those foods knowing the obvious outcome?

That's when the delicate question of "Is it sin?" comes into play. Is it sin to participate in activities that always draw us into destructive behavior even though the activities are not wrong in and of themselves? I can't answer that for you. Each of us has to come to our own conclusion. At the very least, it's unwise to participate in activities that have the tendency to draw us into that destructive behavior, and habitually ignoring the handwriting on the wall is foolish and can be dangerous.

One of the last things I tried before adopting my new lifestyle was one that Nancy read about online, based on fasting nineteen hours a day and eating only within a five-hour time span. I tried it for a little while, actually liking the feeling of fasting so much—as I stated previously, I did live a disciplined lifestyle in many ways, with my longest fast being twenty-one days on water in 1988. And I enjoyed feasting during the five-hour window, timing things properly around my daily radio show or around my preaching schedule on a weekend.

So a little after noon, I would have my first meal (a large chocolate protein bar or chocolate protein shake), then right after the radio show (which ended at 4:00 p.m.), I would go to a restaurant or pizzeria, really enjoying my favorite meal followed by a good-sized dessert, then I was done for the night. And since I'm a late-night person, often staying up until three or four o'clock in the morning, I would be really hungry before going to sleep.

Still, that feeling of fasting was positive (from a spiritual point of view), and I didn't deprive myself when I ate (although Nancy did tell me not to go crazy). The problem was that after doing this for a few days and losing a pound a day initially, the weight loss abruptly stopped, and try as I might, I plateaued very quickly. I was not going to fast nineteen hours of every day for meager results like this! And obviously, I still was not getting the proper nutrition my body needed.

From Nancy: I certainly would not advocate anyone doing this who is not already eating a healthy diet. But this was my husband, whom I loved, and I was trying to help him get that weight off in whatever way I could. It seemed an utter impossibility that he would be willing to change his diet and eat foods he had rejected—with disdain—for decades.

Returning to my pursuit of more energy, one of my friends once told me about an amazing new vitamin containing an energy supplement, but he warned me that it was really powerful (this was somewhere in the early 1990s, I believe). He would take one in the morning and would be flying through the day. I could take two or more and feel nothing. So much for the energy boost.

The same thing happened to me with an amazing grape juice formula guaranteed to cure sickness and boost energy. I drank the allotted amount and, once again, felt nothing. (Apparently there are some health-related benefits associated with this particular grape juice, but for me, there was no energy boost, and that's what I was looking for.)

I also used to buy an energy drink containing large amounts of vitamin C, which I also thought I needed because of the absence of fruit in my diet.[1] One day, my assistant was dropping me off at the airport, and feeling the need for some energy and some extra vitamin C, I drank one of these energy supplements (I might have even have had two of them, if I recall). Then I promptly fell asleep and took a short nap as he drove. So much for the energy burst!

The weight-loss program I enrolled in with the healthy shakes and chocolates also had its own equivalent of five-hour energy drinks, but these were supposedly healthy. The problem was that they didn't seem to work (nor were they that healthy), yet I would try them over and over again when needed. One day they'll give me that needed jolt!

From Nancy: Mike was just unable to make the connection between the foods he was eating and how miserable and exhausted he felt. He was hoping that by adding a vitamin pill or supplement, he would somehow be injected with the energy he so desperately needed. In his mind, there just had to be another way to achieve the results he desired without changing the way he ate, and he certainly tried every ridiculous gimmick.

Sometimes, on long drives when I was tired, I would buy one of those well-known energy drinks (the stronger, the better), and they would definitely help me stay awake, but I knew they weren't healthy long term. In fact, the only products that really did anything for me were caffeine based, and I would sometimes use them to combat jet lag while traveling overseas or to help me push through the night while working on a major writing deadline (which happened fairly frequently). But again, I could tell they weren't healthy—after a couple of days, I could feel the negative side effects—and the caffeine led to more headaches (and other negative symptoms; I'll come back to this momentarily).

One of my favorite stores was GNC, and I'd get the expensive vitamin packs with special energy supplements. Then I'd ask them if they had any new energy-related or metabolism-boosting or weight-loss products—anything I could take in pill form or, if needed, in drink form, even if I had to mix in a powder. But overall, my life remained unchanged. (I'm not saying that GNC has no good products; I'm simply saying the miracle fix never came.)

From Nancy: I can guarantee you, that quick miracle fix is not out there.

On one of my trips to GNC, the guy helping me (who had gotten to know me over the months and was very helpful) suggested I try a great new daily supplement, especially effective when working out. He told me it would boost my energy dramatically—I would feel it all the more during heavy workouts—and it would also boost my metabolism. Talk about killing two birds with one stone!

Well, the first couple of days I did feel quite a difference (this was highly unusual for me, given the way my body is wired), and this exciting new supplement came at a perfect time as I had to write almost every waking hour to get a major book project finished. But by the third day or so, I could tell something wasn't right—have you ever felt that something was messing with your heart?—so I quit taking it shortly thereafter. Of course, I did try it a few more times—maybe the side effects were aberrant?—but then I kissed it good-bye after that. There was a reason you were encouraged to see a doctor before starting to use this particular supplement. (From Nancy: He never told me about this one.)

The simple fact is that *there are no shortcuts to health*, and the most fundamental thing required is a change in our lifestyle: getting rid of the bad foods (rather than just cutting back on them) and replacing the bad foods with good foods (rather than just adding some of them in). Also key is eating to satisfy our real hunger rather than our bodily lusts. Of course, incremental change is better than no change, but incremental change will produce, at best, incremental results, and incremental change will not undo the negative effects of decades of unhealthy eating. And incremental change will not properly purge the body of unhealthy toxins, meaning you will never get completely free from bondage to bad foods with incremental efforts. In contrast, long-term, healthy eating can reverse many dangerous conditions (including clogged arteries and various types of heart disease, type 2 diabetes, autoimmune diseases, and many other serious ailments). And, of course, long-term healthy eating will totally liberate you from destructive food addictions.

The fact is, in every area of life, there are no real shortcuts, including in our walks with the Lord. We can think we're "cutting corners" and avoiding the painstaking, often painful process of real growth, character development, and maturing, but soon enough, our faulty foundations will be exposed. How many times have we seen some young, super-anointed charismatic minister rise up quickly to a place of superstardom in the church, only to have a sudden moral failure and collapse? It's inevitable since the shallow foundation and the lack of deep roots could not sustain the fanfare, spiritual warfare, and fleshly opportunities.

So, as it is with diet fads, so it is with spiritual fads. If you'll give this special offering, your debt will be supernaturally eliminated, despite years of financial mismanagement and carnal spending. If you let the man of God pray for you, your *Not!* knees will be healed, even though your knees are not healthy because of morbid obesity due to decades of unhealthy eating. If you take this new diet pill, you'll lose weight without any effort, while still getting to eat your favorite foods.

I'll say it again: there are no shortcuts to health, be it spiritual or natural health. The Lord is gracious and works miracles on our behalf more than we realize, and it is entirely by His grace that we stand. But that grace also helps us make long-term lifestyle changes, and that's how we run our races with excellence and endurance to the end.

From Nancy: But we like the easy way, the short way. We want to lose weight yesterday! Sometimes, after being overweight for so long and finally coming to the place where we're ready to truly do something about it, we find ourselves at the point where it has become absolutely intolerable—we want to fix it in a hurry. This is understandable. But we cannot lose a hundred pounds in a day, nor can we undo decades of dietary abuse in a moment. But if we make a firm determination to change our eating habits, the weight will come off very quickly, and soon enough we will be looking back from a place of incredible victory.

An additional factor that drove me to change was that, beginning somewhere in the nineties, Nancy and I noticed that I was having problems with my sleep. My ankles and feet would start to twitch once I dozed off, and I would toss and turn through the night, often waking up with the covers off my side of the bed, even the sheets that were under me. Talk about fitful sleep! I was also diagnosed with sleep apnea, ultimately getting to the point where a sleep test indicated it had become severe.

This meant that wherever I traveled around the world, I had to bring my breathing machine with me, and when flying overseas for many hours at a time, I had to try to find a way to plug the thing in (or travel with a battery pack) or else risk having absolutely *miserable* sleep. Added to this was the ankle and leg twitching, which could be maddening during long flights since the twitching would wake me up the moment I started to fall asleep. On one ten-hour flight from India to France, I tossed and turned almost the whole trip (the plane left around 2:00 a.m., so it was bedtime). The entire flight I was absolutely exhausted, unable to use my breathing machine, suffering from a terrible headache, too tired to read or even watch a wholesome movie, twitching myself awake as soon as I fell asleep.

With experiences like this, which were surrounded by day-and-night ministry, you can see why I looked for those magical but elusive health and energy boosts. I was not trying to prove anything with my intense schedule, and I certainly wasn't trying to gain God's favor. I felt (and still feel) loved and affirmed by my Father 24/7. But with a nonstop, unrelenting schedule, I really needed a lift. The gimmicks simply didn't work.

FINDING THE REAL FIX

Today I'm thrilled to say that the sleep apnea has been reduced to very mild, meaning that I don't need to use the breathing machine anymore and that I feel rested when I wake up in the morning. What a relief! Better still, my energy level is off the charts to the point that if I take a short nap in the late afternoon or early evening, I can hardly fall asleep later at night. I still do toss and turn in my sleep and my ankles still twitch, but I'm hopeful that in the coming years that will disappear too. Why not? I'm doing my part, and our God is a healer.

Like everyone else, I still do need my sleep and I do get tired, but it is not a heavy tiredness the way it used to be. And as I mentioned earlier, the headaches, which I used to get three to four times a week, are virtually gone to the point that I've not had a headache (as of this writing) in more than twenty-four months, aside from a mild headache when suffering from some body ache while sick.

Speaking of getting sick, the frequent colds that I used to get are almost a thing of the past, and I can feel my immune system fighting sickness off successfully. The very few times I have gotten run-down and caught a cold after too much travel, not enough sleep, and frequent changes in time zones and climate, the colds are much milder and leave very quickly. I am so grateful to God!

From Nancy: Some time after he changed his diet, Mike told me that it had crossed his mind when he was overweight and suffering such sleep deprivation and exhaustion that he didn't know how long he could keep up his ministry schedule and responsibilities. His enthusiasm was waning. Even though I knew how spent he was, this was a shock to me, and it made me sad to think that the thought of ministry was becoming more of a burden to him than a joy. That sounded nothing like the man I had known for years. It was a reminder that you cannot continually abuse your body decade after decade without paying a price. There are consequences. I used to worry about his health as he was getting close to the age when his own father died of a sudden heart attack (his dad was just sixty-three). Mike had high cholesterol, high triglycerides, and high blood pressure, and was obese. Coupled with the genetic predisposition for heart disease due to his family history, I felt he was a ticking time bomb. But what's a wife to do? Nagging didn't help, and I couldn't force feed him or follow him around on trips snatching the offending foods right out of his hands. That's where prayer came in. God answered and worked a miracle, and I am so thrilled that grace was poured out, enabling Mike to make these permanent lifestyle changes.

Of course, in keeping with my quick-fix health mentality, a mentality I did not hold to in any other area of life, once I started to eat right, I expected to see radical changes in a matter of days, if not a matter of weeks. And there *were* some very positive changes I could feel fairly quickly. But it took a good number of months before I saw real changes in my immune system and, after an initial boost in energy that seemed to level out in those opening weeks, I experienced a dramatic change in my energy level after a couple of months.

As I write these words, I am sixty-one years old. And while I am not boasting about tomorrow and I fully recognize that my life is entirely in God's hands, I am planning to speed up, not slow down, feeling as if I have the greatest and best part of my life ahead of me, and I am very excited to run my race with strength and vigor, by God's grace!

In late February 2016, while speaking near Colorado Springs, Colorado, I asked if there were any guys who wanted to work out with me at my hotel. One man who volunteered to join me was forty and was not in the best shape, so after about ten minutes I suggested he drop out and rest, which he gladly did. The other gentleman was thirty-four, and he ran a lot and even participated in challenging endurance races, replete with obstacle courses and daunting challenges. He also did lots of push-ups and pull-ups in his weekly routine. So he was in excellent shape.

We both did a very challenging workout that my trainer had written out for me, but I had three other challenges to deal with: first, we didn't start working out until 10:00 p.m. Mountain Standard Time, which meant midnight my time; second, I was a little under the weather, clearly fighting something off that week; third, we were at a five thousand-foot altitude, and it's much harder to push your cardio and breathing when you're not used to the thin air.

I told this gentleman I would not push as hard as normal due to having been sick, but I would still complete the extremely challenging workout. To his credit, he fought through to the end, finishing with excellent form. My own form started to break down in the last set of exercises, but I finished in forty-one minutes compared to his forty-five minutes, with hardly any sense of oxygen deprivation because of the altitude. In contrast, in previous years there (or in Denver), I had a hard time breathing in general, at least for the first day or two, and just walking up a flight of steps could get me winded. Now I could do an extensive physical workout for forty-five minutes, starting at midnight and while a little under the weather, all at high altitude. And remember: he was thirty-four; I was a few weeks shy of sixty-one.

From Nancy: Note that this man had the advantage of being much younger than Mike, was not overweight, and was also in good physical shape, yet Mike outperformed him. Why is that? When comparing two brand-new identical cars made at the same factory with the same specs, the one receiving bad fuel will lag and run poorly. But the one with good fuel will run smoothly and efficiently. If we continually put bad fuel in our bodies, they cannot not perform at their peak (and many times cannot perform at all). And really, so much of what we eat could not even be considered fuel of any kind—it's just junk that gums up the works without adding anything to feed and sustain our cells and organs. From a purely health and nutritional perspective, there is no reason to eat the stuff.

For my sixty-first birthday on March 16, 2016, I asked my trainer to give me a workout to do as a test. I wanted to time myself and then use this as a benchmark against which to test myself in future years. He put together a workout with seven exercises, each to be repeated two hundred times, thus totaling fourteen hundred reps, including two hundred jumping jacks, two hundred jump squats, and two hundred wide push-ups. On my birthday, I completed the routine in under twenty-four minutes. Others he was training—including couples in their twenties and in good shape—could not finish it in under thirty-six minutes. This is what happens when you eat for nourishment rather than for indulgence!

Of course, the heavy workouts I do are a great help to my overall health and vitality, but the biggest help by far—really, *the foundation for everything else*—is my totally healthy diet, putting only good fuel into my body.

As for my workout partners that night in Colorado, they were impressed beyond words, with the younger man encouraging me to try one of the endurance tests he had mentioned, where you go through a five-mile obstacle course as many times as you can within twenty-four hours. He assured me I would be tough to beat in my age class.

At this point, I have no intention of accepting his challenge (trekking through mud or navigating sharp fences doesn't particularly appeal to me), and I'm hardly ready to run a marathon (nowhere near it, since I don't run a lot). But I'm in the best overall shape of my life, feeling younger and more vibrant than I can remember. And I'm incredibly excited about the future at an age when many people are slowing down and many others are experiencing serious health setbacks, many of which could have been avoided, sad to say.

One of my dearest friends is an American missionary who has served overseas for more than forty years, primarily in Europe. He and his team major on the majors every day of the week: being disciples and making disciples. They have their daily times alone with the Lord in the Word and prayer, they go to the streets to win the lost during the day, they do outreach meetings at night, and they get new believers plugged into local churches or help disciple them themselves. It's often tedious, difficult work since the harvest is not always ripe, but over the decades they have seen thousands of lost sinners come to faith, and many of them are now in full-time ministry.

Every year, when my friend would come back to the States, he would shake his head at the latest fad—the latest church-growth scheme or the latest secret key to spiritual success or whatever it was—knowing that soon enough, it would make its way over to Europe, only to be replaced by the next quick-fix gimmick. And did any of them produce lasting spiritual fruit? Of course not. As it is with the spiritual, so it is with the natural.

So take it from someone who's been there and done that. The gimmicks don't work and the shortcuts don't produce, from the anti-fat cream to the magic energy pills. Only a radical change in your lifestyle will produce the radical changes you desire, and I can say this without hesitation: it is absolutely worth it!

QUESTIONS FOR REFLECTION

1. Have you tried weight loss or energy gimmicks in the past? If so, see if you can list them. You might be surprised to see the list!

2. Do you tend to look for shortcuts in your life, be they spiritual, physical, or work shortcuts? Have any of them been truly successful long term?

3. Have you consistently prayed for God to give you grace to run your race for the long haul?

4. Are you willing to say to the Lord, "Beginning today, no more shortcuts!"?

CHAPTER 7

MY PLAN WAS NOT WORKING

I N THE LATE 1990s, in the midst of an extremely intense ministry schedule, I put on some weight. I had less time to exercise and my eating habits were bad, as I often ate my main meal late at night, and it was not a healthy meal.

Nancy noticed that I had put on a few pounds and said to me, "I think you've gained some weight."

I replied, "Yes, I did, but I have a plan," and that seemed to satisfy her for the moment.

About six months went by and she said to me one day, "I don't think you've lost any weight."

I replied, "You're right, but I have a plan." And once again, my answer seemed sufficient.

Finally, after close to a year went by, she said to me, "I think you've actually *gained* weight."

I replied, "You're right, but I have a plan," to which she said, "Your plan is not working."

She hit the nail on the head!

My plan—which was really no plan at all, other than thinking that somehow the next day I would do better (perhaps eat fewer peanut M&Ms)—was not working. The next day was the same as the day before. I was deceiving myself, and I was doing it willfully. (Take note of this: you can deceive yourself as easily as you can deceive someone else.)

From Nancy: Let me be clear. I was not deceived and understood full well from day one that he would not be losing weight. But I didn't want to become a nag, so I let it ride.

Fast forward to August of 2014, when I was as heavy as I had ever been. Nancy was never under any illusion that my plan would work and had really been praying about my weight, being concerned for my health and knowing that my blood pressure had been rising over the years. I had been praying as well, being embarrassed at my obesity (although hardly anyone, except Nancy, would have thought I was ninety-five pounds overweight) and realizing that I couldn't play games with my health as I approached sixty years old in the midst of a very heavy life schedule.

As Nancy and I talked that day, I said to her, "My plan is not working." And that was the beginning of the breakthrough.

I finally accepted the fact that more of the same would only produce more of the same, and I knew that, despite losing thirty pounds or more a few times in my life, I was steadily gaining weight over the years and was fatter than I had ever been. If I was to be honest with myself, I would have to admit that there was no way my incremental changes would produce the radical results I needed.

Many years earlier, I had given up sweets entirely, but that lasted a matter of months rather than years. And my times of special discipline—such as eating sweets once a month—petered out after a while as well. I had cut out fried foods most of the time, and I didn't eat a lot of red meat. But the truth be told, I had way too many fried chicken tenders, way too many french fries, way too many steaks, and way, way, way too many unhealthy desserts—not to mention those endless pizza slices.

My plan was not working, and I knew that I had to make a dramatic change and that I needed Nancy's help to make that change. And so, when Nancy said to me, "Starting tomorrow, I want you to eat only what I give you," I knew I had to comply. This was the grace of God at work, and when our Father is kind enough to intervene in our lives, we need to seize the moment. I am profoundly grateful to the Lord for stepping in.

From Nancy: I told Mike that if he gave me complete control over everything that went into his mouth, I could guarantee that he would lose weight and lose it quickly. His high blood pressure would go away, his high cholesterol would go away, all his blood work would be normal, and he would have more energy than he knew what to do with. I was surprised he agreed to let me take control in this way (and was inwardly jumping up and down!). He was not allowed to eat anything that I didn't provide for him, and he could only eat the specific amounts I prepared. He didn't have to think or make any decisions about what to eat. All he needed to do was ingest what I set before him. He definitely looked a little scared.

I'm not a control freak, and it certainly wasn't my desire to be master over my husband, but he genuinely wanted help, and I knew he didn't have a clue how to eat properly. So in the area of diet I was going to think for him and make all the proper choices. It was a little tricky because I had to devise ways to sneak his most despised foods into the meals I prepared for him. But with God's help, I was able to do it.

Of course, at that point I didn't realize I would be doing this the rest of my life—I couldn't have handled the thought at that time—and I still had some things stashed away in a cabinet in case I got desperate (some jelly beans if I needed something sweet, because I was determined not to have anything chocolate other than a chocolate protein bar, which I ate the first two mornings as I got started). But once I got going and broke free from those miserable food addictions (see chapter 9), I realized that I was being supernaturally empowered and that, by the incredible love of the Lord, I was being saved from a premature death and granted a fresh, healthy start. (I'm not being presumptuous in any way, and my life is entirely in His hands. Only He knows what the future holds. But I'm quite sure that healthy eating leads to a longer, healthier life and unhealthy eating leads to a shorter, less healthy life.)

I never did touch those jelly beans (I got rid of them), I never had another chocolate protein bar, and as of this writing, more than two years later, I am not looking back for a split second. My plan was *not* working, this better plan *is* working, and with the help of God, this is the plan for me. I've also found that remembering that "my plan was not working" is a great help in times of temptation, which were more frequent in the beginning and are almost nonexistent now.

The fact is that I really enjoy eating the way I eat today, but because I'm on the road all the time, I'm eating at restaurants on a regular basis, and the people taking me out to eat are often ordering the foods I used to eat. And those foods can still look good, meaning I can be faced with potential food temptations on a regular basis.

Only a couple of months into my new lifestyle I was ministering in Hungary at the largest megachurch in Europe. A member of the congregation is a top Italian chef now based in Budapest—he used to cook for the prime minister of

Italy—and on my last day there, he was catering a private meal for us. Talk about some nice-looking pasta with some sumptuous red sauce and mozzarella cheese! (No, I didn't have a single bite, but my salad was great.) The opportunity was there, but there was virtually no temptation. Why? I had been there and done that, and my plan didn't work. Simple.

When I fly business class overseas, there are some delicacies that I enjoyed having for years—for some reason, I craved the pretzel rolls on some flights, not to mention the special sundaes they would make for dessert, along with the endless chocolates and cookies—and then there are the many hours spent in airports. I knew in each terminal where the Sbarro's pizza was or where I could get chocolate yogurt with Oreo toppings or an Auntie Ann's pretzel, and often, because of the timing of my flights, the only time I could get a meal was at the airport. I had all my special eating places mapped out at every airport around the world.

And then there are the many trips to the grocery store, passing the familiar seductive aisles with all my old, favorite treats. They often looked good to me, especially in the early days of healthy eating. I should also mention that my wonderful mom, ninety-three years old as I write, has a real sweet tooth, although she's as thin as a rail and quite frail (but very sharp mentally). So I am often shopping for her too, which means getting her the chocolate cookies, dark chocolate kisses, chocolate truffles, and other chocolate candies she so loves, not to mention the gummy bears and crystallized, sugar-coated ginger.

As I walk those grocery store aisles, gazing at the ice cream section (those double-chocolate Magnum bars look so luscious); as I sit at those really nice restaurants, observing what others devour at the table (a chicken parmesan dinner at Carrabba's Italian Grill still has its appeal); as I breathe in the smells at the airport (hey, I was never into Cinnabon, but it does have quite the aroma), I say to myself, "I tried that, but my plan was not working." And just like that, the spell is broken. The lie has been exposed.

I've been there and done that, and it didn't work for me.

Case closed.

Temptation ended.

From Nancy: I knew I needed something in written form to remind me of how important it was to me that I reach my goal. I seem to forget that when temptation is there. All I'm thinking about is how good that doughnut will taste going down, forgetting that when the stupor is gone and reality hits, it won't feel good at all. In fact, it will feel terrible—and the terrible feeling of regret will far overshadow the good taste of the doughnut one hundredfold.

But even knowing that, somehow when my favorite food delicacies are staring me in the face, I strangely lose all remembrance of the misery I feel being overweight. It's as if I'm in a trance or someone wiped the memory of what happened just an hour before when I was trying to squeeze into my jeans (the jeans that really didn't fit anymore). How could one little doughnut have the power to control my thoughts and erase my memory? How could a doughnut cause me to forget that I will regret eating it? (I always regret it, so why can't I remember that?) Why don't I remember that I'm going to wish I never took that first bite to begin with? And why can't I remember the sense of joy and relief I'll feel after I've chosen not to give in. Such a wonderful feeling and I can never seem to remember it.

It's a strange thing, the power of food addiction to wipe out the memory. To stand strong in the face of temptation, I needed a reminder, something in my own words that could convey all the emotions connected to being overweight (the desires and regrets in all their intensity) and snap me back to reality, because for some reason none of that exists when that doughnut is calling me. So I made a reminder for myself, a list of all the ways overweight and food addiction has hindered my life, and all the things it has prevented me from participating in—a list with all the accompanying emotions. It's a substantial list with many tentacles, very sobering and not necessarily pleasant to read. But it's a useful tool and has the power to break the spell of doughnuts and wake me up to reality.

But it's my list, and if needed, you will have to make your own, because only you know the depth and intensity of the destruction overweight has caused in your life. The tricky part will be having enough discipline to pull that list out and actually read it when all you want to do is eat. Sometimes, strangely enough, we avoid taking our medicine, even when we know it has to ability to fix what ails us.

It's best to pray before we're in a place of desperation. Continually pray for strength and grace so it will be there even before you find yourself in need of it.

DON'T PLAY GAMES WITH YOUR DELIVERANCE

The rewards of the new life are so wonderful and the downfalls of the old life so miserable that, to repeat, I'm determined never to go back to my old ways, with the help of God. My old plan didn't work back then, and it surely won't work the older I get. I can't imagine going back to being fat, going back to feeling sluggish, going back to high blood pressure, going back to using a CPAP machine for sleep apnea, going back to backaches and headaches. Why in the world would I want to do that? Yet the vast majority of people who lose weight gain it right back plus more. Why is that?

From Nancy: Many regain their lost weight because they have the diet mentality. They haven't made a permanent lifestyle change, and when they lose the weight and the diet is over, they go back to their old way of eating—ingesting the same foods that made them fat in the first place. This hardly ever works and statistics prove this out. (See point number one in chapter 15 for some specific examples of this.)

Think about it in light of the principle of Matthew 12:43–45 and 2 Peter 2:20–21, which states that it's worse to go back into bondage after being set free than it is to be in bondage in the first place. The last state is worse than the original one. Applied to food, this would suggest that having been set free by the Lord in such a wonderful way, should I go back to my old ways of eating, it would be much worse in every way: I would gain more weight, it would be harder to take the weight off again, it would be very difficult to get back on track and stay on track, and the negative health consequences would be more acute. The lesson is simple: *never play games with your deliverance.*

I believe there's also a physiological side to this. I've read that when you gain weight repeatedly, things happen within your cellular structure that make it more difficult to take the weight off. We actually gain more fat, and we gain it more quickly too, and our body composition changes. We are working against ourselves tomorrow when we indulge the flesh today.

One day at the airport, just trying to find an apple, I spotted one of my all-time favorite snacks, one that I sometimes I had a hard time finding at many airports: a decadent, fudge-covered brownie with walnuts. In fact, in the past, when I did find one at an airport, being a spiritually minded man, I almost felt like the Lord had provided it for me as a special blessing. (For sure, when I would get to a hotel to check in after a long journey and there were those free, fresh-baked chocolate chip cookies at the counter, I was almost sure those were a gift from heaven. I'll talk more about this in chapter 9.)

On this particular day at the airport, I could not find a single healthy thing, and when I finally spotted an apple, it was right next to those brownies. I looked at it and said to myself, "Yes, it looks really nice, just like an attractive woman I'm not married to, but it's off limits, just like that woman." There was no more possibility in my mind that I would eat that brownie than there was the possibility I'd try to pick up another woman. The very thought of it was as absurd as it was distasteful.

That's how I look at these other foods. They're off limits for me, and the more time that goes by, the less appealing they look. Those unhealthy foods are totally detrimental, contrary to all my goals, and with nothing good to offer. Really now, is it worth sacrificing your health for a temporary food high? Is it worth having a bulging belt line in order to indulge your flesh for a few short minutes?

Think about it for a moment. Did you ever pig out until you couldn't eat any more and say to yourself, "I'm so glad I did that!"? On the flip side, did you ever say no to a food temptation only to feel so good about your decision the next day?

From Nancy: I never regretted denying myself unhealthy, tempting foods. Maybe I did at the very moment when the struggle was flaming, but afterward, when I was in my right mind, I was thrilled I hadn't given in and relieved that I didn't have to wait until the next morning to start life all over again. But quite the opposite was true if I yielded to temptation. The day basically ended there. It was a failed day—a wasted day—and I couldn't get rid of the cloud that had descended on me until I woke up the next morning and started fresh. I always try to remind myself about the feeling of disappointment I experience after taking that first bite (and what inevitably followed after).

It is really the rarest of times that I feel tempted at all, and I truly enjoy the foods I eat. But when temptation comes or I feel a little deprived—after all, most of the people I'm with are eating unhealthy foods, and some of them outwardly appear to be healthy and some are even thin—I just remind myself, "I've been there, I've done that, and it didn't work for me." My old plan wasn't working, the new plan is working wonderfully, and it will work wonderfully for you as well.

Maybe this is your breakthrough moment when you finally confess, "My plan is not working!"

Why deceive yourself any longer? A new life is knocking at your door and you only have to answer yes—leaning hard on the Lord, but with the recognition that you have no other choice. He, on His part, will not let you down. What will you do?

From Nancy: Through the years, I lost and gained weight several times and tried different diet plans, all of them extreme and unhealthy. I've gone on high-protein, low-carb diets that have the potential to damage the kidneys, increase the incidence of heart disease in susceptible individuals, and have been linked to premature death, as documented by Dr. Fuhrman in his books *Eat to Live* and *The End of Dieting*.[1] I also followed severe low-calorie diets that caused my hair to fall out in massive amounts, and I've been on several other extreme, unbalanced eating plans that landed me in an advanced life-support ambulance on my way to the hospital because of a potassium deficiency. (It took me more than a year to regain full strength because I was so depleted. Thankfully, there was no long-term damage, but I could have killed myself.) And of course, I always gained all the weight back.

I did learn my lesson, though, and never repeated my folly, but it left me not knowing which way to turn when I was finally ready to make a change. Unfortunately, many people following some of the diets that are currently popular are unaware of the health risks associated with them. They think they're fine because an online doctor with an attractive website said so, and that if so many people are following it, it couldn't be bad. Unfortunately, with most of these diets, there is no concrete scientific evidence to back up their many claims (although they might cite a study or two, they fail to mention there are four additional studies that disprove or contradict their conclusions). I've learned you have to do your homework thoroughly and cannot believe everything you read, especially online (even if it comes from someone with an MD after his or her name). You will find that all solid research confirms the benefits of a well-balanced, plant-based diet.

QUESTIONS FOR REFLECTION

1. Have you tried weight loss plans in the past? If so, which ones? And what were the end results?

2. Are you living in denial in terms of your own weight problems?

3. Do you recognize that you need a whole new lifestyle and a fundamental change in your relationship to food if you are to see lasting change?

4. Have you confessed to the Lord (and to others who want to help you lose weight), "My plan is not working!"?

CHAPTER 8

HOW MY RADICAL TRANSFORMATION BEGAN

WHAT WAS IT that triggered the radical transformation in my life beginning August 24, 2014?

Often it takes a crisis to spark a radical change, but sadly, in many cases, once the crisis comes, it's too late to change course or make the needed corrections. Too much damage has been done, which is why it's best to make the radical changes before the crisis. That being said, if it's a crisis that is causing you to read this book now, don't despair. God is a redeemer, and it may not be too late to turn things around in your own life.

From Nancy: It's really extraordinary to see the dramatic transformation that healthy eating can produce. People who were just steps away from bypass surgery or whose diabetes was out of control, and many who spent thousands of dollars on medications and health care have had their lives totally turned around and transformed by changing their eating habits. It's not a pipe dream, and the ability of the body to heal itself is an incredible thing to see. God has created something truly amazing. If we just cooperate with the way the Lord designed things to work, we'll be stunned by the results.

In my case, in one sense there was not a crisis, but in another sense there was a crisis. Allow me to explain.

There was *not* a crisis because, overall, I was in relatively good health. My body was functioning well, I kept a vigorous personal schedule (including, as I mentioned, lots of travel around the world), and I could do grueling physical workouts with men one-third my age. My mind was sharp and my body was not breaking down (at least not that I could see), and although I was obese, most people didn't think of me as being obese—just a tall, somewhat heavy guy.

On the other hand, there *was* a crisis. For years, my cholesterol levels had been marginally high (based on our somewhat loose American standards; based on more rigorous standards, they were high, period), which meant that for decades there was the potential that my arteries were getting clogged. More ominously, my blood pressure was rising, reaching a high of 149/103, and that meant I clearly had hypertension (high blood pressure), which is called "the silent killer."[1] You don't play games with a silent killer!

You can see from this chart how high my blood pressure was.

Stages of High Blood Pressure in Adults[2]

Stages	Systolic (top number)		Diastolic (bottom number)
Prehypertension	120–139	OR	80–89
High blood pressure Stage 1	140–159	OR	90–99
High blood pressure Stage 2	160 or higher	OR	100 or higher

Rather than waiting until your next doctor's visit, may I strongly encourage you to invest thirty dollars and buy a blood pressure cuff so you can take your own blood pressure at home? If you're afraid to check your blood pressure out of fear of negative results, then you really need to go out and get that blood pressure cuff today. Don't stick your head in the sand.

For years Nancy kept one of these blood pressure machines at home to check our blood pressures, but as I got heavier and was working out a lot, we had to buy a larger one because my arms were too big. And I was actually proud of this! "My muscles have really grown," I thought to myself. Once I lost my fat, I fit into the original cuff with ease, and my biceps and triceps today are actually fairly large and well-defined. It was the fat that didn't fit into the cuff, not my muscles.

So although outwardly I was fairly healthy, there was a potential crisis looming under the surface. But that's only part of the story. The truth is, I hated being fat, even though virtually no one (other than my sweet wife) ever said anything to me about it, and even though, to this day, most people who knew me back then say, "But you were never that heavy." But I was! I weigh between 180 and 185 pounds now, and at the highest, I weighed 275 pounds. That is obese, plain and simple, and it was dangerous.

Although I never talked about it publicly, I was embarrassed by my weight gains over the years, even when I weighed 225 or 240 pounds. In my mind, this was not in harmony with how I lived my life as a disciplined servant of the Lord willing to make sacrifices for the gospel and saying no to the flesh and the world every day of my life. Why, then, was I overweight? Why couldn't I say no to chocolate or candy or unhealthy snacks or unhealthy meals?

For years I had lied to myself saying, "Tomorrow will be different," but except for rare stretches of time (like the late summer of 2000, when I got down to 215 pounds for a few days, and this right after a three-day fast), my plan was not working and tomorrow was no different than today (see chapter 7 for more on this). Worse still, as the years went on, little by little, I was getting heavier, and for the first time in my life, my "fat clothes"—those clothes I wore at my heaviest—were starting to get tight. (Most of us have clothes like that, don't we?) My waist now is 34 inches. At my heaviest, it was at least 44 inches, probably 46, but I bought the relaxed fit, stretchy jeans to avoid the harsh reality. When I was at the heaviest weight of my life, under no circumstances was I going to buy fatter clothes.

From Nancy: Obviously, a healthy lifestyle isn't all about vanity; it's about taking care of the body God gave us and fueling it properly. But certainly, our appearance does come in to play. For me, getting dressed and trying to look halfway presentable as a fat person was an exercise in futility. It's very hard to hide layers and layers of fat and feel good about yourself. I would wear the same old dark-colored "thing"—I called it my uniform—whenever I would go out to social functions, which was rare. I would drag myself into my closet and try on more articles of clothing than I could count, only to emerge wearing that same old dark, potato-sack-like "uniform."

I was much more obsessed with my appearance as an obese person than I am as a thin person. Now I can put on something and not be concerned about the way I look at all. I don't even have to look in the mirror. I feel good and look normal, and don't feel like the fat outcast (which is how I always used to feel). I'm not horrified when I see my reflection in a plate-glass window or concerned that I have nothing to wear. And I'm not afraid to get on the scale anymore. My life is just wonderfully, blissfully normal.

Most of us realize that as we get older, our metabolism slows down, and so if we eat the same size meals we ate when we were younger, we'll put on weight. And since we tend to be less physically active the older we get, we put on even more weight. For me, not only was this the case, but every year, either during the holidays or during a family vacation, I would eat extra for a few days and put on some weight, then never take that weight off. So, little by little, I got to a place I never thought I'd be. In fact, I simply wouldn't get on the scale because I didn't want to be discouraged.

I would look in the mirror and think to myself, "You look like a slob!" I would be around other leaders who were not heavy and say to myself, "If you're really a man of God, why are you the heaviest person in the room?" And when I was not upgraded to business class or first class on long flights, those airline seats were starting to get uncomfortable, leading me to ask myself, "What's next?"

Thankfully, the moment I would start to minister, my only focus was on the message and the people and the Lord, and so being overweight never once hindered me from preaching, teaching, debating, or standing for the truth. But many others don't feel the way I did about being fat, and they are so embarrassed by their obesity that they are paralyzed by it. It can be a real confidence-killer to say the least. I know some people who won't even leave the house because they are so ashamed of their weight. Nancy was this way when she was overweight.

For me, while the breaking point came in August of 2014, things had been building for years in terms of both extreme tiredness (or frequent, minor sickness) and growing embarrassment about my weight. To cite just a few examples out of many in my journal, on May 1, 2004, I wrote, "Another good day of teaching (9:00–4:00), but physically, I am in terrible shape, still dealing with some kind of allergies, still totally wiped out and tired, still having great trouble redeeming the time. Abba! How can I effectively serve You and advance Your kingdom when I'm wasted like this?" Then, on June 12, 2004, this entry: "If I could only get some rest. My sleep has been so interrupted, so fitful, despite my breathing machine. This is really wearing on me." Six months later, on December 11, 2004, after playing some intense rounds of Ping-Pong, I noted how I got "easily winded when I really push," adding, "I *will* get in shape!"

On February 5, 2005, after pushing too hard and getting run-down, I wrote how Nancy was concerned "that my health will simply not hold out." I continued, "I owe it to my bride—along with the Lord and those He has called me to touch—to get into the best possible physical shape. I do want to run my race to the end! (And how can I run so as to win if I don't 'finish' the course?)"

These were constant themes in my journal over the years. For Nancy, who has an incredibly accurate and totally uncanny ability to see where there is a problem and to identify where something is going to go off track, her greatest concern was not my appearance but my health. Of course she wanted me to be a good witness for the Lord, and that included me not being fat, but much more importantly, she knew the health risks of obesity. She knew that the fat I was carrying around my stomach and chest was potentially deadly. And she knew that high blood pressure was not something you could play with.

That's what drove her to prayer for me in August 2014. And so, as I was crying out to the Lord in one part of the house, unknown to her, she was crying out to the Lord in another part of the house, unbeknownst to me.

But let me return to my journal entries for a moment. On February 6, 2005, the very next day after the last journal entry I just cited, as I read about significant Christian leaders in their seventies and eighties, I wrote this down: "What is God's purpose for me in this generation? How many of the burning, massive dreams in my heart will I live to see realized? Right now, the big issue for me is ongoing tiredness and the need to get into vibrant health and press in to the Lord more deeply. The rest is in His hands—which is good enough for me."

On March 16, 2005, I turned fifty, and I wrote: "This year, my deepest requests are: 1) Greater personal discipline to draw deeper in spiritual intimacy and to get into good physical shape (and finally take off this excess weight for life)....Can I see running this race for thirty more years? Why not? Unless I'm called to lay down my life as a martyr, there's no reason that I can't believe for good health, work toward good health, and stay focused and productive for the long haul, even if the pace will eventually change a little." You can see how these issues were on my mind at that time.

Then on April 28, 2005, while praying late at night about all the things that were bothering me in life and ministry, these were some of the entries toward the end of my long list (they were still heavily on my mind despite their placement on the list): "11) My weight....13) My constant tiredness, despite my efforts to use the CPAP [breathing] machine, to eat better...I would be so much more effective in God with more energy and strength! And being tired, it's easier to be lazy, since I don't want to push too hard for a number of good reasons. And how miserable it is to be starting a new trimester next week [teaching at FIRE School of Ministry] when I'm feeling the need for a vacation!"

Fast forward almost ten years, and things were worse, not better, as reflected in these entries: December 31, 2013: "My goals for 2014 (not surprisingly): ...lose 50 lbs. By God's grace!" Then March 25, 2014: "I am so bothered by my weight and I'm finding it so hard to be disciplined in diet on the road (and, less so, at home too). By God's grace, I must make some radical changes. Just eliminating sweets (and/or snacks) wouldn't really do it." Then August 11, 2014: "I am so bothered by my fat!"

And then this entry, the day before I began this wonderful, new, blessed lifestyle: "Nancy was really praying for me today, asking God for ways to help me with my diet, and I know I have to make radical changes."

So my faithful bride was earnestly seeking God on my behalf, knowing that I could not continue living the way I was living, asking God to give her creative ways to cook things for me that I would be willing to eat, knowing my terribly limited taste preferences. On my end, I had reached my fat limit, so to say (as I mentioned I was *not* going to buy any bigger clothes). And as I looked ahead to my schedule in the coming months, which included speaking at some of the most significant congregations in the world and recording a series of meetings that would be broadcast on international TV, there was only one thing on my mind—and it was *not* the messages or the schedule or the travel. It was my fat.

That month, August 2014, I was talking with my son-in-law Ryan as we walked around a carnival where we had taken some of the kids while on vacation in Maryland. I said to him, "There's only one thing on my mind before these meetings, and it's my weight." He was surprised to hear it.

During that vacation the grandkids were playing in the pool at the hotel, so I put on a pair of gym shorts and a dark T-shirt and got in the water with them. (I didn't have a bathing suit with me and I wasn't going into the pool without a shirt on, not just out of Christian "modesty" but also because of my weight.) Our older daughter, Jennifer, was taking pictures, and when I saw what I looked like in that soaked T-shirt, I was shocked. How in the world did I get this big? That was one more push in the right direction for me, and it was not a gentle push. It was a real wake-up call.

A NEW LIFESTYLE

And so I too cried out to the Lord for help, and when Nancy and I talked together on August 23, 2014, for the first time in my life (as I shared in the last chapter), without excuses and without equivocation, I said to her, "My plan is not working." She replied, "Just eat what I give you to eat." Knowing that I had to make the change, I agreed to start the next day, little realizing that it would become a lifestyle.

How grateful to God I am for my amazing friend and companion of more than forty years, the ideal match for me in this world—and how grateful we both are to the Lord for His miraculous intervention, since it was nothing less than that. He moved on both of us to pray, He answered our prayers, and He helped me to do something that had seemed impossible for me until that moment in my life—or so I had thought. To repeat what I've said throughout this book, He will do the same for you if you cast yourself on Him and do what you're able to do.

There was one more factor that brought me to the crisis point, even though, as I stated, in other ways there was no crisis. I know the promises God has given me for my life, and to the best of my knowledge I have barely scratched the surface of what He has called me to do. So even though I've seen amazing things over the years and even though I've packed enough into this one life to fill three or four ordinary lives, I am constantly looking forward to what is ahead. Yes, I firmly believe that the best is yet to come!

The problem though was that I was getting more and more tired as the years went on. How then was I supposed to run my race with perseverance to the end? How was I supposed to run my race so as to win? (See Hebrews 12:1–4 and 1 Corinthians 9:24–27.) How could I continue doing two hours of live radio daily, write three to five new articles a week, put out one or two new books per year plus keep up my scholarly writing, travel two to three weekends per month and go overseas at least five to six times per year, teach weekly at our ministry school and serve as a professor at other seminaries, produce new TV shows, respond to endless e-mail requests, be a mentor to others, spend quality time with my family, have intimate time with the Lord—how in the world could I keep up a schedule like this? I was getting older, not younger, and something had to give.

Of course, I recognized that at some point in time I would have to cut back on certain activities, but I didn't feel the time for that had come. Plus, when you're more tired, you're less excited about the things you're doing. So in 2014, for the first time in my life, I started to get just a little burdened by the thought of years of heavy ministry ahead. In the past I was always excited about the future.

I can tell you now that by God's gracious help, I feel younger than I have in years, I am constantly exhorting people less than half my age to keep up with me, and I am absolutely stoked about the future. I *know* the same things can happen to you if you too will say, "Enough is enough! The time for change is now."

From Nancy: Feeling tired and run-down can certainly cause discouragement, but eating poorly and being nutrient deprived can also have a direct effect on our mental well-being. Eating highly refined, processed foods with lots of sugar and additives affects our brain chemistry and can lead to depression along with intense highs and severe lows, especially after a sugar-fest (similar to drug use). I was always surprised by how tired and down I felt after waking up the morning after a night of eating lots of chocolate, cake, or cookies. It felt like I was on Nyquil. It's amazing how eating a clean, healthy diet can keep us on an emotionally even keel.

So this is some of what was going on in my life when God brought me to that point of radical change. And while I certainly wish I had the made change earlier, I am blessed beyond words to find myself where I am today.

Let me leave you though with one word of wisdom. By all means, make your resolution to change today, and certainly, if the Lord is putting His finger on any area of your life, respond to Him right now. But take your next steps wisely. Finish reading this book and then if you want to know exactly how Nancy and I live and understand why eating the right foods—and not just cutting down on portions or getting rid of the worst foods—is so important, get Dr. Joel Fuhrman's book *The End of Dieting*. Between our book and his, you'll have all the motivation and information you need to lead a truly blessed, health-filled life. How wonderful it will be! (There are other healthy, plant-based eating plans out there that are very similar to Dr. Fuhrman's, and any of those plans will work.)

Whether you follow the Fuhrman plan or another healthy plan, take some time before the Lord and tell him, "Father, I recognize that I'm fearfully and wonderfully made and You have made me a steward over my health and my body. I want to glorify You with my body and live my life to the full for You. Give me the grace to walk in discipline, help me to resist unhealthy eating just as I would resist any other sinful temptation, and give me a vision of how my life can be changed by changing my relationship to food. In You I am an overcomer!"

Begin to picture yourself thin and full of vitality. It is certainly God's desire for your life, and when it comes to making changes like this, without a doubt He is for you, not against you. Surely that is enough!

QUESTIONS FOR REFLECTION

1. Are you facing any health problems right now? If so, are any of them related to unhealthy eating?

2. What's the number one reason you are reading this book? Do you have sufficient motivation to make a radical lifestyle change, by God's grace, beginning today?

3. Do you feel that unhealthy eating could rob you of experiencing many of the promises of God? Is it worth it?

4. When is the last time you saw yourself as thin and full of energy and life? Why not take some time to ask the Lord to give you a fresh vision of this?

CHAPTER 9

BREAKING THE FOOD ADDICTIONS AND REPROGRAMMING MY MIND

S UNDAY, AUGUST 24, 2014, was the first day of my new lifestyle. That morning, before speaking at my home congregation, FIRE, I still kept my old habit of eating a chocolate protein bar, but from then on, I was only going to eat what Nancy gave me, beginning with a big salad and a bean pasta dish. This was a first for me, but it was an idea Nancy got while praying about how she could help me change my eating habits. So I ate the pasta dish made from beans (which was topped with a healthy red sauce), and I enjoyed it somewhat, even though it was different. It didn't look like normal pasta, it didn't taste like normal pasta, and it didn't quite feel like normal pasta (yes, texture matters, doesn't it?). But the sauce was good, even if it had some extra items I didn't like that much. So far, so good.

Nancy also told me that I was allowed a carefully rationed portion of raw, unsalted nuts and seeds every day (cashews, pistachios, sunflower, and pumpkin, which are very healthy and an important part of any diet). I was allowed fruit, and then there was a chocolate substitute treat later—a very small brownie made from black beans, cocoa, and dates, with some cut up walnuts and cashew cream topping. It was pretty good too—today it's a delicacy—and I made it through the day without cheating.

Having these healthy substitutes was a tremendous help to me (I don't think I could have made the transition without them, and the healthy pasta idea came to Nancy in answer to her prayers). There are actually lots of healthy substitutes for unhealthy foods; there are recipe books with many options.[1] Over time, you'll find them totally enjoyable and satisfying—without the guilt or negative side effects—although at first they taste nothing like their unhealthy counterparts. You'll also find that these healthy substitutes—without sugar, fat, and salt—are self-limiting and not addicting, meaning you don't desire to stuff yourself with them. You might want to have another portion, but the desire stops at a certain point.

From Nancy: When I told Mike that he was permitting himself to eat only what I gave him, the pressure was on because I had no idea what to feed him. He had an aversion to most of the foods that are good for you, so I really cried out to the Lord to give me some ideas. The trick was getting the foods he disdained into his meals without him noticing, since if he knew they were there, he wouldn't be able to get the food down. He liked pasta—that was one of his favorites—but white pasta was out, so I thought I'd try "bean" pasta (there are some good ones out there). I believed if I put enough sauce on it, that would be sufficient to disguise the texture, flavor, and look of it.

I concocted a plain marinara sauce and ground up

mushrooms (they have lots of health benefits) in a food processor until they looked a bit like a pâté. Ground this way and cooked in a sauce or soup, they basically disappear. You can't see them or taste them (I even used this trick on myself when trying to learn to eat mushrooms). I also snuck in finely chopped broccoli and kale along with many other healthy items (all chopped so minutely as to be unidentifiable). And since Mike loves onions (which are also healthy), I heaped them on. That first meal was a complete success—he didn't vomit or hate it; he even liked it a little. Although I prayed that God would work a miracle and intervene, I was still somewhat surprised that it actually worked and Mike was willing to continue! Thankfully he enjoys eating tomatoes and tomato products—that makes it easy to hide just about anything in all different kinds of soups and stews. In appendix D we have included a list of helpful resources, including some cookbooks.

That first night of my lifestyle change, I journaled, "I have grace, but I don't find this easy. Despite really lagging at night, wrote two articles."

By the next day, I was feeling miserable—and I mean miserable. The toxins were leaving my body, and it was not fun at all. *Yuck!* I also had a mild cold, and doing my live radio show for two hours was a real chore. I continued to eat the right things only—I forget what meal we experimented with; the very large salad was the biggest part of my eating—but I felt really lousy all the time. The relevant part of journal entry for the day read: "Day two of my healthy eating regimen, struggling to be focused as the junk is leaving my system (no doubt that I have lots of food addictions)....Breaking my food addictions is challenging!"

The misery continued throughout the third day, but I had

read enough to know that bad stuff was leaving my body—poisons, really—so as miserable as I felt, I understood that it was a good thing. Addictions are not broken easily, and I had more than my share of food addictions, especially sweets. I also realized that at some point in time I was going to have to go through this, so now that I was three days in, I had to see it through. But it was getting really tough!

Late that night I cried out to the Lord in prayer, reminding Him of how real Jesus was to me when He set me free from drugs on December 17, 1971—the night I promised the Lord I would never put a needle in my arm again—and how I had been free from that night on. I asked Him with fervor and passion to be so real in my life that I could break free from my chocolate addiction for life as well. Surely the Lord who delivered me from heroin and other drugs could deliver me from chocolate!

But to be perfectly honest, breaking free from chocolates and other foods was harder for me than breaking free from drugs. The food addictions felt stronger than the drug addictions (I was addicted to the needle and to drugs in general; I was not a heroin addict) and the withdrawal from addictive foods was worse than the withdrawal from drugs. "My Father and my God, help me again!" I prayed.

This was my journal entry at the end of the third day: "I feel out of it in every way: so tired and groggy, despite a good night's sleep, plus with cold symptoms still. Radio is fine despite the way I feel, play cards with my [then ninety-one-year-old] mom, then pray for a bit by the pond behind her building, teach night class (the counterculture revolution of the 1960s, with video footage that shakes the class up, as always), home to answer e-mails, then try to be productive late and have a breakthrough in fervent prayer for deliverance from food addictions."

Under the special category of Prayer Requests I wrote:

"Father, I am very weak when it comes to food—my mind is weak and I've never eaten healthily for a prolonged period of time my entire life—and I confess my inability. So, just as *You* delivered me from heavy drug addiction and from Diet Coke and sodas, I'm asking *You* to deliver me from my bad food habits and change me into a healthy-eating man."

God answered my prayer that night! After three days of detoxing, the withdrawal symptoms were gone, never to return. Some people go through this for five or even seven days (or longer), but either way, as long as you keep filling your body with healthy foods (I'll discuss this more in the last chapter), the misery will soon end and you'll start feeling the positive results of healthy eating.

But do you really have a choice? If there are deadly snakes in your basement, do you just leave them there, or do you hire an exterminator and get rid of them? If there's a deadly leak in your ventilation system, do you simply tolerate it as it slowly kills your family, or do you a hire a specialist who can get to the root of the problem and correct it? Why then do we allow deadly poisons to reside in our own bodies? Why do we allow harmful toxins to downgrade our health and reduce the quality of our lives? And why do we tolerate unhealthy addictions in our bodies?

From Nancy: In the Old Testament God called the Israelites to annihilate the Canaanites—not to have mercy on them, not to intermarry with them, not to spare them. You don't play games with a deadly problem. For Israel to spare the Canaanites was to seal their own doom. God said to Israel: "When the LORD your God brings you into the land that you are entering to take possession of it, and clears away many nations before you, the Hittites, the Girgashites, the Amorites, the Canaanites, the Perizzites, the Hivites, and the Jebusites, seven nations more numerous and mightier than you, and when the LORD your God gives them over to you, and you defeat them, then you must devote them to complete destruction. You shall make no covenant with them and show no mercy to them. You shall not intermarry with them, giving your daughters to their sons or taking their daughters for your sons, for they would turn away your sons from following me, to serve other gods. Then the anger of the LORD would be kindled against you, and he would destroy you quickly. But thus shall you deal with them: you shall break down their altars and dash in pieces their pillars and chop down their Asherim and burn their carved images with fire....And you shall consume all the peoples that the LORD your God will give over to you. Your eye shall not pity them, neither shall you serve their gods, for that would be a snare to you" (Deut. 7:1–5, 16). If food is a snare to you—meaning that it is destructive and is hurting your life—treat it ruthlessly.

HOW TO DETERMINE IF YOU'RE A FOOD ADDICT

You might be wondering, "Well, how do I know if I'm addicted to certain foods? I never thought of it like that. Or what if I'm just plain addicted to food?"

In *The End of Dieting* Dr. Fuhrman offers this checklist of fifteen questions to determine whether we are food addicts:

1. If I don't eat regularly, I feel fatigued or irritable. Yes or No

2. I think about eating certain foods almost all the time. Yes or No

3. I feel sluggish or uncomfortable after eating.
   Yes or No

4. Eating poorly is interfering with my health.
   Yes or No

5. I'm overweight, but I continue to overeat.
   Yes or No

6. When I start eating sweets, I don't want to
   stop. Yes or No

7. I have tried to diet to lose weight, but failed
   and given up. Yes or No

8. I prefer restaurants with all-you-can-eat buffets.
   Yes or No

9. I have physical withdrawal symptoms.
   Yes or No

10. I sneak food when others aren't around or
    looking. Yes or No

11. I store food or hide food from my family.
    Yes or No

12. I eat more even though I'm no longer hungry.
    Yes or No

13. My eating habits cause me distress. Yes or No

14. My eating habits are causing me social and
    family difficulties. Yes or No

15. I eat almost continuously all day long.
    Yes or No[2]

Did any of those apply to you? One? More than one? The majority? Well, brace yourself. According to Dr. Fuhrman, "One 'yes' answer makes you a suspected food addict. Two or more 'yes' answers confirm your addiction to food."[3] Ouch! This suggests most of us are food addicts, perhaps seriously so.

One easy way to test whether you're addicted to a particular food or a specific way of eating is to go without that food (or change the way you eat) for twenty-four to forty-eight hours. Were you able to go the distance? If not, that answers the question right there. If so, did you find yourself craving that food or that way of eating (meaning not just thinking, "I'd like to have that," but actually feeling a need for it)? Did you find your body reacting to the absence of this particular food (or to its absence at a specific time of the day)? Did it affect you emotionally? If so, you're probably addicted to a particular food (be it chocolate, like me in the past, or coffee or fried foods or whatever) or to an unhealthy lifestyle (late-night junk food snacking or gorging yourself), and the only way to get free is to make that dreaded (but so wonderful) radical change.

A headline in October 2013 announced: "Student-Faculty Research [at a Connecticut college] Suggests Oreos Can Be Compared to Drugs of Abuse in Lab Rats."[4] According to an article from the school's website, "Connecticut College students and a professor of psychology have found 'America's favorite cookie' is just as addictive as cocaine—at least for lab rats. And just like most humans, rats go for the middle first."[5] I could relate!

The article continued:

> In a study designed to shed light on the potential addictiveness of high-fat/high-sugar foods, Joseph Schroeder, associate professor of psychology and director of the behavioral neuroscience program, and his students found rats formed an equally strong association between the pleasurable effects of eating Oreos and a specific environment as they did

between cocaine or morphine and a specific environment. They also found that eating cookies activated more neurons in the brain's "pleasure center" than exposure to drugs of abuse.[6]

No wonder I found it harder to get off sweets than to get off drugs. And no wonder so many Americans are serious food addicts. The fact is that *many of the foods we eat on a daily basis contain ingredients that are addictive.* Peanut M&Ms are no longer my friends! Double-Stuf Oreos no longer have a place in my life! They are enemies, meant to enslave me and harm me, and the momentary pleasure I used to get from eating them is not worth the long-term pain.

This may sound radical to you, but can I ask you honestly: are you free or are you addicted? If you are sure you have no food addictions—be it to sweets, meats, breads, or anything other than healthy vegetables and fruits—then go completely cold turkey from your favorite foods for one week (or one month). Maybe you're not as free as you thought you were.

But breaking free from the physical addictions is only the first part of the journey. Mental strongholds must also be broken, and in many ways, these can be even harder. The good news is that we are not slaves to our minds, and especially as believers, we can renew our minds and change our whole way of thinking.

During those first few weeks, Nancy would send me a testimony every day from someone whose life had been *dramatically* transformed by healthy eating (specifically, following Dr. Fuhrman's *Eat to Live* guidelines),[7] complete with before and after pictures. Some of the stories were almost hard to believe. A 300-pound man on multiple medications who was scheduled for heart surgery and barely able to walk around his house without getting exhausted now weighed 160 pounds, had completed his third marathon, was free from all medication, and had avoided the heart surgery. And all this in less than two years!

If these people could do it, I could do it, especially since some of them were not believers and made these dramatic changes entirely by their own willpower. Surely with God's help, I could make similar changes. Plus, my situation was not so dire: I was still in relatively good health, I worked out heavily, and I wasn't quite as overweight as some of these other people. I could have a great testimony too!

Nancy would also send me great quotes from Dr. Fuhrman, who is a real no-nonsense guy. These quotes would hit me between the eyes in a positive, life-giving way, further motivating me to do what was right. (One I remember said, "You will never fulfill your life goals if you are chronically sick or dead.") But as I took these initial steps, I quickly realized that the biggest strongholds were in my own mind, and for me, food was my reward. Allow me to explain.

BREAKING MENTAL STRONGHOLDS

In February 2016 Nancy asked me to watch an episode from the TV series *My 600-lb Life* that told the story of a young woman, married with a child, who weighed 725 pounds and now realized she did not have much time to live without making radical changes. It was painful to watch—my heart really goes out to people who are so dangerously obese—but it was very informative, which is why Nancy wanted me to see it.

I was aware, of course, that people overeat for different reasons and not just out of lust for food or because of addictions. Some eat for comfort. Some eat as a way of escape. Some eat when they are frustrated. For the poor woman in this program, she ate to find comfort and to mask her pain, a habit she developed after she was sexually abused as a little girl and then continued to be abused to protect her sister from abuse. Her father was not there and her mother, addicted to drugs, was there in body only. And so the one place of escape this little girl found, the one place where all was well and her world was secure, was the place of food. Now she was killing herself with eating—she knew it and shed many tears over it—but it was food that gave her comfort in her pain. So the thing that helped her emotionally was killing her physically. What a terrible trap!

Some of you can relate to that fully, even if you don't weigh 700 pounds. Others can relate to it in part since we think to ourselves, "I know this is bad for me and I'll regret it tomorrow, but it tastes so good and I really want it!" For this woman, though, the bondage was severe, and breaking her bad eating habits after getting stomach-reduction surgery solved only part of her problem. She had to change her whole way of thinking, living, and even feeling.

What is interesting is that once you make a radical life-style change, you will quickly discover the role food plays in your own life. For me, food was my reward, and there were food associations that colored almost every area of my life. Take away my favorite foods, and everything felt different and empty. How could there be joy without those treats?

I began to analyze my thoughts and focus on the nature of this stronghold in my life. (Remember, the issue was not going without food. I was getting enough good food— huge amounts, really—to meet my body's needs every day. The issue was not getting to eat my old foods.) I would get dropped off at my hotel after a rigorous preaching schedule and now it was time to unwind—and that meant special food treats. It was time to heat up that bag of microwave butter popcorn, put some sports on TV, then munch on chocolates and relax. I deserved it! And if I hadn't eaten before the service, I might order in a pizza before the snacks.

But food wasn't just my reward after lots of public speaking. It was built into the very fabric of my life. As I mentioned earlier, at the major airports that I frequented, I knew which one had Auntie Anne's pretzels, which one had Sbarro's pizza, which one had Ben & Jerry's ice cream, which one had gourmet burgers—you get the picture. And because I was on the road, I was therefore *allowed* to eat this. (And I was on the road a lot!) This was one of the perks.

It was the same while flying. On domestic flights I would normally get a free upgrade because of my frequent-flyer status, and that meant free snacks, such as pretzels, nuts, and sometimes Milano cookies. It would be wrong to refuse *free* snacks while flying! As for traveling overseas on long flights (some as long as fifteen hours, sometimes followed by another eight-hour flight), I would do my best to use my frequent-flyer miles to upgrade or else try to get a discounted business-class fare, and that meant much better food (along with the vastly better seats, which was the main reason for flying business class).

Certain flights had my favorite rolls (pretzel rolls and cheese rolls), other flights featured a custom-made vanilla sundae with chocolate sauce and nuts, and some flights offered unlimited snacks, including Oreos, European chocolates, or other sumptuous dainties. And they were free for the taking throughout the flight. How could I pass up a blessing like this? When I arrived at the hotel, there would often be freshly baked chocolate chip cookies at the reception desk. I would take two or even three, eating one immediately and saving the other(s) for later. (I liked to put them in the refrigerator, enjoying them cold.) What a gift from God!

From Nancy: That's quaint—eating just one complimentary cookie and leaving the rest for later. This is a completely foreign idea to me. I could eat an entire bag of cookies (I meant it when I said I ate enormous quantities of food). One bite of most of my former foods would keep me wanting more and more of that good taste. If I ate one cookie, I would want another one and another and another.

I wanted to duplicate that good feeling—that dopamine rush—but each time I ate those highly palatable foods, I needed more of them to give me that same feeling. You have to continually eat larger and larger quantities of the offending foods to get a sense of satisfaction. For me, there was no such thing as, "I'll have a little taste now and save the rest for later." That's laughable. I could eat an entire 12-ounce box of pasta along with almost an entire stick of butter, heavy cream, and parmesan cheese in one sitting, and then crave something sweet for dessert.

There were also the special perks of being in different cities. Back in New York I had my favorite pizzerias and Italian restaurants, while in Chicago I knew the best places for deep dish pizza. Overseas there were lots of amazing meals. In Korea there were restaurants with delicious bulgogi, cooked right there at your table; in India there was butter naan and garlic naan and chicken tikka; in Italy—who can describe the wonders of Italian cuisine, including those balls of Buffalo mozzarella cheese doused in special oil and seasoning, with some fresh basil leaves to top them off? From the homes where I was entertained to the restaurants to the hotels, the Italian cooking was exquisite, a blessing from heaven, for sure.

From Nancy: Mike ate for his reasons. I ate all the time for all reasons. I ate when I was happy. I ate when I was sad. I rewarded myself for a job well done. I celebrated special occasions with food. I ate if I was under stress. I ate when I was relaxed. I ate when I was tired. I ate when I was rested. The only time I lost my appetite was when I was afraid, which obviously didn't happen that all that often.

Back in the States, in my normal day-to-day life, things were no different. Food treats were the perk that made everything special, and the absence of those perks took the fun out of everything (at least that's how I felt when I started confronting these mental strongholds). Why take the grandkids to a fun family movie if I couldn't share popcorn with them and then munch on a box of chocolate nonpareils? Why watch a sports event with friends if I couldn't eat my favorite snacks? Why go on vacation if I couldn't eat freely every day? Why go on a long drive if I couldn't stop at the convenience store and get an assortment of munchies? And on and on it went.

Of course, the reason I would go on a long drive (or take a long flight) was to get somewhere, but without special food perks there seemed to be no reason to go. And the reason I'd take the grandkids to a nice clean movie was to have fun with them, but without the special snacks it didn't feel like fun—at least that's how everything felt to me when I contemplated it. That meant that with God's help, I had to renew my mind and change my whole way of thinking. Food was the fuel for my life, and the joy of life was not found primarily in food but in life in the Lord.

I remember one of those early days when I had first changed my lifestyle. I was thinking back to the time before I was a believer, for some reason daydreaming about the rock concerts I attended as a teenager. Suddenly the thought hit me, "But how could I enjoy those concerts without food?"—after which I immediately said to myself, "But I didn't eat at those concerts!" (It's true I went to the concerts high on drugs, but the fact is that I didn't associate rock concerts with food.)

What I realized was that somehow in my thinking, almost

every enjoyable thing I did had an associated food perk with it, and on a daily basis there was special anticipation for my pizza (or other special meal), then for the chocolate treat that would follow (although I sometimes said to myself as I bought a candy bar at the grocery, "Aren't you acting like a little child?"), then for the food rewards I would give myself as I wrote through the night and into the early morning.

Not only was I constantly feeding carnal appetites, but I was also living to eat rather than eating to live, to the point that life without food treats didn't feel like life at all. How utterly shallow and silly—and yet that is how many of us live, as if life is not enjoyable without unhealthy food.

Perhaps your eating patterns are very different than mine, but whatever they are, to the extent you can identify your own particular stronghold, to that extent you can effectively take those thoughts captive and ask God to fill any of the voids. Then you can begin to eat to live rather than live to eat. (For practical steps for breaking these strongholds, see Nancy's story in appendix B.)

I still do enjoy my daily meals, and I enjoy healthy snacks while hanging out with the family or while taking long trips. But my attitude is totally different than it used to be, and I can assure you that I am *thriving* in every way. Life is more than food!

QUESTIONS FOR REFLECTION

1. What one food do you most dread giving up? Tell your Father about it right now. He won't condemn you or mock you.

2. Has the Lord set you free from other sins and addictions in the past? Do you believe He can set you free from food addictions too?

3. Do you know the primary reasons you eat unhealthily? Addictions? Love of certain foods? Comfort? Frustration? Anger? If you think about not eating the foods you love most, you will be able to see what else is attached to those foods in your thinking and your emotions.

4. Do you unconsciously think that life is not worth living without eating what you want when you want it? Can you even imagine a wonderful, new life that is full and overflowing without unhealthy eating? If even imagining this new, healthy lifestyle seems impossible, ask the Father to deliver you from this stronghold of hopelessness and give you a vision of yourself enjoying eating healthy foods.

CHAPTER 10

"I CAN'T! I CAN'T!"

I REMEMBER THE NIGHT vividly.
It was Tuesday, September 9, 2014, and I had returned home after my daily radio broadcast to catch a short nap before teaching my night class at FIRE School of Ministry.

I was now fifteen days into my new lifestyle, and on this particular day when I woke up from my nap, I was feeling very hungry—or, more specifically, I felt an intense craving for food, in particular, something sweet.

From Nancy: Mike was always claiming hunger, and I would tell him, "You can't possibly be hungry; you just ate dinner." But he always insisted he was hungry. He would be nibbling and munching and chewing all night. And he seemed to have amnesia about it. The problem was, he didn't really know what true hunger was, and most of us don't. We're so in the habit of eating for the sake of eating or just for pure pleasure. If we learned how to respond to our body signal of genuine hunger, the amount we put in our mouths would be cut in half.

Now I had read in a nutritional book that having a sweet tooth was a good thing since we needed healthy sweets like fruits in our diet. But this craving felt intense, not healthy, and I wasn't exactly craving an apple. What was I to do?

There was no way I was going to get a piece of unhealthy, sugar-laden chocolate—by God's grace that addiction (as opposed to the desire) had been broken after three days, and I was only looking forward, not backward—but for some odd reason we had no fruit in the house, and I had only a few minutes to spare before leaving to teach. So I got in my car ,and on the way to school I stopped at a convenience store, hoping they would have some cut up watermelon. (To be candid, until just a few days before this, the thought had never once entered my mind to look for watermelon at a convenience store. But I had actually seen some in one of those stores that same week, hence the thought of looking for it again.)

From Nancy: Don't confuse addiction and desire. They're different. The alcoholic who goes through detox has now broken his body's physical addiction, but there's still an emotional and mental desire for the alcohol. It looks pretty in the glass and has an appealing aroma. The mind remembers the warm feeling the drinking brought (though it conveniently forgets the destruction that came along with it).

So even when the addiction is broken, the lure can still be there. I know people who are completely repulsed by the old foods they used to eat. They don't look appetizing to them anymore. But that's not the case with me! Those foods look incredible and smell amazing, and I would love to eat them. And to be honest, I'm not sure the attraction will ever go way. It might, but if not, I'm prepared to deal with it.

Mike and I completely stay away from unhealthy

foods. We can learn how to respond to enticement. As I mentioned previously, I had to write down all the negative fruit of overeating—physical, spiritual, and emotional—and I read it when I'm facing temptation. If you ask Him, God will show you how to set boundaries and resist the foods that tempt you most. And when He does, it will just take practice and a bit of resolve to walk it out.

That night, to my disappointment, there was no watermelon and no other fruit, so I began to look at the available fruit juices, knowing that in general they were off limits for me because of the sugar content and other artificial ingredients. But the craving was intense, and I had to do something, so I found some Naked juices (that's the brand name) and looked for the healthiest ingredients I could find. (Nancy says I'm not the biggest whiz when it comes to knowing what healthy ingredients are.) I then drank half the bottle before class, and that's where I hit my breaking point: a complete, momentary emotional collapse. (Go ahead and laugh at me as you continue to read. I was actually watching myself from the outside laughing—really—as I broke down crying in my car.)

I suddenly felt overwhelmed. *I cannot do this!* I cannot live the rest of my life under this kind of pressure. I cannot live the rest of my life without ever having another slice of New York pizza or another piece of chocolate or another dish of ice cream. I cannot live like this! And right there, sitting in my car outside our school building with literally one minute before class, I cried like a baby saying, "I can't! I can't!"

As I said, this whole episode really is laughable (if not downright pathetic), and as I broke down crying—as in *crying with tears*—I was actually watching myself, laughing at the spectacle, as I cried like a baby in my car. At the same time I knew it was all for the good since I needed to come to the end of myself in order to enter into God's strength. As the Lord said to Paul (in a very different context!), "My grace is sufficient for you, for My strength is made perfect in weakness," in response to which Paul said, "When I am weak, then I am strong" (2 Cor. 12:9–10, MEV).

On the one hand, I had lived a disciplined life in many ways for years, and so I was used to saying no to fleshly desires on a daily basis, including desires for certain foods (or certain amounts of foods). On the other hand, this new lifestyle really was too much for me. I needed the Lord's supernatural grace.

You see, in almost sixty years of life I had never lived the way I was living. I had never eaten the new foods I was eating and never abstained from all the other foods I had eaten for decades, some of them on a daily basis for years. To live like this for the rest of my life—that's a long time—seemed like a burden too heavy to carry, especially given my intense ministry schedule and high-pressure lifestyle. In fact, that's what hung me up in the past whenever I tried to take off weight: *I could not live with the constant sense of being deprived.*

It was enough for me to take up the cross on a daily basis and say no to the flesh in general—to live a holy, counterculture lifestyle in obedience to the Lord—without adding in dietary deprivation. In reality, I *enjoyed* living under pressure, with constant flights to catch, constant writing deadlines to complete, constant speaking engagements to fulfill, constant spiritual attacks to fend off. I was born for battle, and I felt grace to run the race the Lord had called me to, and that included going against the grain of the world and swimming against the tide of the flesh.

But there was a limit to all this. For example, when my ministry is under financial pressure (this has happened more than once), it feels oppressive, calling for more leaning on the Lord in prayer. And in the past when I would cut back radically on my food intake—substantially reducing my calories, abstaining from all sweets, or whatever the change would be—this was the straw that broke the camel's back. Too much pressure!

I simply could not take the added weight of feeling deprived all the time—and I mean all the time. There was that minor gnawing I felt day and night when I had dieted in the past, that desire for more food, that feeling that something was missing physically, that sense of *dullness*, almost like a bleak, overcast, rainy day where the sun never shines. That's how life felt when I made serious changes to my diet. And now I was making a total, complete, absolutely radical, lifetime change. "God, I can't!"

THERE'S NO COMPARISON

I quickly wiped the tears from my eyes, and as I was getting out of my car, the Lord laid it on my heart to change the direction of my class (just for the record, the class had nothing to do with food or diet), and it turned out to be the exactly right topic for the night. How gracious our Father is!

More importantly, that was the night everything changed, and from that day to this, now more than two years later, I have never had a food crisis again, not even once. Here and there, on the most minor level, while walking through an airport between flights looking for something to eat—it's not easy to find something healthy at the airport—I'll have the *slightest* feeling of deprivation, almost feeling sorry for myself. But this is very rare, it is very brief, and it's easily dispelled. I am thrilled with my new lifestyle, and everyone who spends time with me, in particular those of my own generation, envies me for it.

Who can compare a bag of potato chips with a vibrant, thriving healthy life? Who can compare the momentary pleasure of a thick, luscious milkshake with a glowing report from the doctor? Who can compare a big, juicy steak with boundless energy and years of additional, energized living? And what would your family say if they could have you around for an extra five, ten, or twenty years, healthy, strong, and vigorous? Would the sacrifice be worth it or not?

But there's more. I *love* to eat apples now. I *love* eating my giant dinner salads. I *love* eating the healthy chocolate replacements Nancy makes for me (using things like dates for sweetness). I even *love* the pseudo-pizzas I cook up once a week (using Ezekiel bread pitas, a healthy, organic red sauce; some healthy pseudo cheese; then some toppings such as onions, tomatoes, or basil). It's all delicious!

As for the foods I don't like as much, I still enjoy eating them since they're still satisfying, and above all I know they're providing the needed fuel for my full and intense life. And since your taste buds really will crave whatever you feed them, why not feed them healthy things? Even if it took a month or two (or more) to reprogram your palate, wouldn't it be worth it for the years that would follow?

"But that's the whole problem," you say. "I've tried to do it over and over, and I always end up failing."

That's exactly why I wrote this chapter. Sometimes we need to come to the Lord and cry out for a breakthrough from of a place of weakness. Sometimes we need to acknowledge our weakness.

"God, I confess that I'm a food addict. I confess that my stomach is my god. I confess that I'm lacking in willpower and that I've tried to lose weight and get in shape too many times to count. Help me, Father, and demonstrate Your strength through my weakness!"

If you're sincere and you really desire to change, and if you're genuinely willing to make a radical lifestyle adjustment, God *will* help you. You might go through some times of desperation, feeling hopeless, times of crying in your car, as I did, as if your prayers are not getting through. But if you will keep crying out, the breakthrough will come. After that it's up to you to realize that in Jesus you are an overcomer. In Jesus you can live a disciplined life. In Jesus your flesh will not rule. Instead, you will rule over the flesh. And the longer you do the right thing, the easier it will be to do the right thing and the harder it will be to go back to the wrong thing. It really will become a new lifestyle, and the more you live it out, the more you will enjoy living it out.

Don't forget that plenty of other people have made this radical shift, and many of them have done it without prayer, faith, or supernatural intervention. They simply had enough with unhealthy living and determined to restructure their lives. Years later they are healthy and strong. Surely with the Lord's help you can do it. Surely your body can thrive by living the way our Maker intended us to live. If they could break through, you can too.

The big key is that you can't just make some minor adjustments if you want to see dramatic and long-term change. As many leading doctors have demonstrated, the standard American diet—which is high in sugar, salt, and unhealthy fats—is deadly. And if you want to see real, lasting results and want to be a good steward of the body God has given you, you'll need to think in terms of serious lifestyle adjustment.

Are you willing? Then keep reading.

QUESTIONS FOR REFLECTION

1. Do you feel powerless to change your eating habits? Do you feel defeated by food? In Jesus you are an overcomer!

2. Have you learned the power of leaning on God in the midst of your weakness? Do you

understand the scriptural principle of, "When I am weak, then I am strong"?

3. Have you hit bottom before in your life—losing all hope—only to see that your extremity was God's opportunity? How can that experience apply to your struggles with food?

4. Have you understood the confession of, "I can't do it in myself" to be the beginning of, "In Your power and by Your strength, I can do all things!"? Then your very first step is to keep reading until you finish the book and follow the recommended guidelines in the last two chapters.

CHAPTER 11

BLESSED WITH THE GIFT OF BEING "ALL IN"

A FEW MONTHS INTO my healthy eating lifestyle, I was getting a physical exam at my doctor's office. He's a fine Christian as well as a terrific doctor, and we've gotten to know each other a little over the years during office visits. As we discussed the radical changes that had taken place in my life, he remarked, "You're blessed with the gift of being 'all in.'" He was absolutely right!

Before I knew the Lord, I was heavily into drugs and rock music—and I mean heavily. I spent almost every free moment listening to rock music, playing rock music, going to rock concerts, and getting high. On the music side, I was considered the best rock drummer in my school. On the drug side, I was considered the heaviest drug user in my school (in terms of large doses of drugs) to the point that I earned the nicknames "Drugbear" and "Iron Man." (This is shameful and nothing to boast about; I'm simply sharing my history.)

Once I was born again and developed a solid relationship with the Lord, if I wasn't attending a church service or doing evangelistic work or fellowshipping with my friends,

I was reading the Word (at least two hours a day), memorizing Scripture (twenty verses a day), or praying (at least three hours a day). This was all before I started working a full-time job or going to college, so I had more free time on my hands. But I zealously used that free time to meet with the Lord, and by His grace I made every hour count. I think you can easily see what my doctor meant when he said I was "blessed with the gift of being 'all in.'"

From Nancy: I think it's important to understand that Mike is not a superman since you might be thinking to yourself, "Yikes! This guy memorized twenty verses a day, as well as praying three hours daily; no wonder he can make these radical dietary changes. He's different." The fact is that he has the same struggles everyone else has (trust me on this) and needs to stay disciplined in the Word and prayer and resist the flesh just like the rest of us. In Mike's early years as a believer, God chose to give him an unusual, supernatural season where he had many free hours to pray and read the Word, enabling him to memorize thousands of scriptures. But it was no easier for him to change his eating habits than anyone else. He needed God's grace just like we all do.

The Lord set me free from shooting drugs on December 17, 1971, and from that day on I never put a needle in my arm again. Two days later I renounced all drug use and was free from that day on. (This is all by His grace!) So I went from being totally in to totally out.

Somewhere around 2004 the Lord began to convict me about my Diet Coke habit (I'm not saying this is sinful for everyone; God simply convicted me of it.). I was definitely addicted to it and was drinking at least three to four 16-oz. bottles a day. Once again by God's grace I was able to break the habit fairly easily, and from that day on I've never had another sip of it. In fact, since Diet Coke was the main soda I drank, once I stopped drinking it, I basically gave up all other soft drinks, instead having only water, sparkling water, or seltzer (carbonated water).

When I was in college, I got really interested in languages, starting with Hebrew. At one point I was studying Hebrew, Arabic, Greek, Latin, German, and Yiddish, all at the same time. (By the way, this is not the best way to learn new languages!) Then when I went to grad school for my master's and PhD, I added a few more languages, mainly ancient Semitic ones. Yes, when I go for it, I go for it.

This mind-set has been a tremendous help with my new lifestyle—once God helped me make a break with my old ways, I did it with all my heart, not deviating from the path one iota. In other words, I never eat anything unhealthy. No exceptions. Ever. I'm all in! And when people say to me, "How often do you cheat?" I reply, "How often do you cheat on your spouse?" (Of course, I'm not comparing committing adultery to having a Snickers bar. I'm simply saying that if something is wrong and off limits, it's wrong and off limits, be it a little or a lot.)

From Nancy: People slip and fall all the time. Not everyone is like Mike in this regard. Some people hit a lot of bumps along the way, and it takes them awhile to find their stride. So if you commit to a healthy lifestyle and mess up two days later, don't throw in the towel because "Mike Brown did it without messing up." We're all different, and some of us might fall numerous times before we find long-term success. The point is to pick yourself up and keep going and not let one failure stop you. As the Word says, "For the righteous falls seven times and rises again" (Prov. 24:16). We all have our strengths and weaknesses, and I can assure you

that Mike has his weaknesses too. But there was a lot
of prayer that went into this, and so God poured out His
grace. Remember to pray!

Now you might have a totally different personality than I
do—perhaps the exact opposite of my personality—but when
it comes to lifestyle changes, I want to commend to you the
"all in" mentality. It will save you a lot of grief and jet-propel
you into success. In fact, if your mentality is, "No exceptions, ever," you'll find that after a while you're hardly ever
tempted to eat poorly since the possibility doesn't even exist
in your mind. Not only so, but you'll reap the best results
from healthy eating, since a little bad food can undermine
the full benefits of a lot of good food.

I WASN'T ALWAYS THIS WAY

To be perfectly honest, though, I didn't start off with this
"all-in-for-life" mentality when I began eating healthily. No
way! That would have been way too hard for me to accept.
Instead, Nancy and I often talked about when I would
have my first cheat day and what I would eat. Would it be
after three months? Maybe one slice of pizza? Or would I
go six months? Maybe a steak? Playing these mental games
helped a lot, and Nancy gave me a great line to use whenever I felt tempted: "I can eat whatever I want, just not today."
Psychologically, it worked!

From Nancy: When I started to eat healthfully, I determined to be all in (I'm an all-in kind of person), and
I was going 100 percent, no exceptions. After I felt
pretty set and secure in my eating habits and had lost a
good deal of weight, I thought it would be OK for me to
have a very limited, controlled, and thoroughly planned-

out cheat day once a month. That's exactly what I did—with disastrous results. The disaster wasn't immediate but happened over time. I thought I was strong enough to eat some of my old, unhealthy foods and then just go right back to eating the healthy foods again. But all it did was stoke my appetite for the things that had been so destructive to me in the past. And the new healthy foods that I had come to really enjoy were now completely unappetizing to me. If you treat yourself to Godiva chocolates, how appealing is a stalk of broccoli going to be after that? It's not—at least it wasn't for me.

The very next day after my cheat day I had no desire for healthy foods. I forced myself to eat well, and after a day or two my "healthy" appetite came back and I loved my greens again. But each time a cheat day came around, it became more difficult to go back to healthy eating and took much longer to enjoy the good foods again. And one cheat day became two and then three. As difficult as this is to accept, wisdom dictates that for me, there are no cheat days. It just doesn't work.

As time went on, the more I ate healthy foods, the less I needed to play these games, and today a "cheat" day for me—say, on my birthday—is to eat as much *healthy* food as I want, such as extra nuts or healthy crackers or healthy sweets. Although I've indulged myself like that a few times, I don't enjoy it that much since I don't like to feel full. Plus, on the positive side, there are some healthy foods, especially salads, that you can eat in large quantities every day (with healthy dressings, of course), so you end up eating a much larger volume of food than you normally would.

I have also learned the difference between toxic hunger—when your body is deprived of unhealthy, addictive foods and your stomach growls or you get a headache or shakes or feel weak (most people think this is a sign of hunger, but it's actually a sign of withdrawal from the addictive, toxic foods)—and true hunger—when your body wants some healthy nourishment. I'm also doing my best to avoid snacking (whereas in the past I snacked all night long) since it becomes mindless, unnecessary, largely unhealthy eating. And when you snack, you never learn to listen to your body's real signals for food. This too required discipline before it became a way of life.

At this point you might be thinking, "Forget about it! I could never live like this, not even for a week, let alone for a lifetime. I'll just deal with being fat."

But you're missing something really important: every day you live like this, you're making progress. The weight starts to come off automatically (how good is that?) and you start to feel so much better physically, emotionally, and perhaps even mentally. Those old clothes that you couldn't fit into for years start to fit you just right, and some of your chronic illnesses are disappearing as well. You really start to feel great, and the foods you eat are quite satisfying and enjoyable. I'd say it's a pretty good deal after all!

But here's the essential point I want to make: It's all too easy to blow it. It's all too easy to get off track. And just like a former alcoholic who's been sober for twenty years can fall back into alcoholism with just one drink, the same could happen to you or me with food. Why give it a chance? Why open the door?

Maybe you're the type of person who could "cheat" one day a month for life and never more than that. There are still downsides to that (as I mentioned, the little bit of bad food lessens the full impact of all the good food), but if that's who you are and that's how you live, fine. I just don't think that's the case with most of us, and if I can splurge on my birthday, why not on our anniversary too (in our case, those dates are just two days apart, so maybe I should splurge for three straight days). And if I can splurge on Thanksgiving, why not on Christmas too? And what about on our daughters' birthdays or the birthdays of our sons-in-law or our grand-kids? And what about when we have a special church gathering or I'm taken to a fancy restaurant or I'm in a foreign country where I can get a very special, one-of-a-kind meal?

If I say it's OK for me to cheat once every six months, who's to say that won't become once every three months, then every month, then every week, then every day? Before I know what happened, I've gained back all the weight I lost (that would be a horror) and undone all the good I did. May that never be, Lord!

There are many people whom Nancy and I have been acquainted with who lost lots of weight through healthy diet plans but then totally "backslid" in their eating habits and put their weight back on simply by opening the door just one time. (I'm sure you know people like this too.) To say it again: Why give it a chance? And is it really worth it? The real tragedy is that many of these people were not able to get back on track again once they messed up. Why play with fire?

Proverbs gives this stern warning: "Can a man scoop a flame into his lap and not have his clothes catch on fire? Can he walk on hot coals and not blister his feet?" (Prov. 6:27–28, NLT). If food has been your downfall, then you can apply these verses to eating wrong foods. Why play games with something so dangerous?

Again, you might be the type of person who can "cheat" a little here and there with no negative consequences. That's between you and God (although it's a bit of a hard sell if you're fifty or hundred pounds overweight or suffering from lifestyle diseases such as high blood pressure, heart disease, or type 2 diabetes). As for me, when I'm at the airport during a long layover, watching people eat all the foods I used to eat, I say to myself (especially when some of those eating unhealthy foods are very slim), "Maybe they can do that, but I can't. Maybe they can get away with that occasional slice of pizza, ice cream cone, or burger and fries, but I can't."

The truth is that I lived like that for decades, and it was *not* an occasional splurge but a daily splurge (meaning that virtually every day I ate something unhealthy). As I said in a previous chapter, my plan was not working, and the reality is that I was getting fatter and unhealthier by the day. There was no happy medium for me, and I see no reason to experiment with the gracious help the Lord has given me. And for what? For a momentary food pleasure? For something I'll regret the next day? For something that might trigger old addictions? For something that might even make me sick? For something that might not even be enjoyable after so much healthy eating?

But there's something else that needs to be said. *No one really gets away with unhealthy eating.* Yes, I've seen the stories of people who lived past a hundred and who ate unhealthy meals for decades (actually, for ten decades!). But they are the rarest of rare exceptions to the rule, although I used to point to them as proof that I didn't need to change my diet. The fact is that there are people who are slim but still unhealthy, people who seem to be doing fine but drop dead of a heart attack, people who could be much healthier and live much longer if they ate healthier.

Why not then go "all in" on healthy eating? The benefits so far outweigh the drawbacks that it makes perfect sense. And the reward of occasional "cheating" does not outweigh the risk of falling back in your old, destructive eating habits.

So I'm not here to judge you or tell what you do. I'm simply here to commend the "all in" lifestyle and to say that when it comes to a healthy lifestyle, there's no such thing as too much of a good thing. And if by God's grace I continue to live like this until I leave this world and meet the Lord, I'll gladly take the risk of Him saying to me, "Son, you were a little too hard on yourself. You could have eaten a brownie once a year."

That's a risk I'll gladly take, especially when food in the world to come will presumably be better than anything we ever had here on earth, but without those fattening, addictive, and deadly qualities. So I'll enjoy all the benefits of healthy eating and living while here in this world. And it is my hope that I'll produce many more fruitful and focused years of service to the Lord and others. Then I can feast in the world to come. The fruit of the tree of life should be sumptuous!

QUESTIONS FOR REFLECTION

1. Are you "all in" when it comes to following the Lord? Are you willing to be "all in" when it comes to healthy eating?

2. Are you able to receive forgiveness if you initially fall short of your goals? It's important that you don't condemn yourself if it takes you a little while to get fully on track.

3. Do you know others who were doing well in their lives—be it in healthy eating or freedom from substance abuse or some other newfound liberty—only to fall back to their old ways after they opened the door just once? What can you learn from this?

4. Would "cheat days" be playing with fire for you?

CHAPTER 12

THE ESAU MENTALITY
IS DEADLY

H E WAS ONLY forty-eight years old when he dropped dead of a massive heart attack last night, and his family is in complete shock. Devastated would be a better word. Why did he die so suddenly? And why at a time like this, just five days before he was scheduled to walk his oldest daughter down the aisle and give her away in marriage? Now, rather than joy, there will be agony, and the wedding will have to be postponed because of all the funeral arrangements. "Daddy, why did this happen?" the eldest daughter sobs.

Although this particular scenario is imaginary, similar stories, equally tragic, occur every day, leaving behind a sea of tears, years of pain and mourning, children without a parent, and spouses without their beloved life partner. What makes these stories all the more tragic is that when it comes to heart disease, the vast majority of these tragedies could be avoided. Even in cases where the heart disease is allegedly hereditary, what is often "hereditary" is bad eating habits, and even when there are real genetic propensities toward heart disease, healthy eating could prevent those diseases from ever developing, even with those who are predisposed to them.

Do you remember what Esau did in Genesis 25? The text states:

> Once when Jacob was cooking stew, Esau came in from the field, and he was exhausted. And Esau said to Jacob, "Let me eat some of that red stew, for I am exhausted!" (Therefore his name was called Edom.)
>
> Jacob said, "Sell me your birthright now."
>
> Esau said, "I am about to die; of what use is a birthright to me?"
>
> Jacob said, "Swear to me now." So he swore to him and sold his birthright to Jacob. Then Jacob gave Esau bread and lentil stew, and he ate and drank and rose and went his way. Thus Esau despised his birthright.
>
> —Genesis 25:29–34

There is an abrupt feel to the Hebrew in verse 34 describing Esau's activities, as if in a moment of time he gulped down his meal and sold away his birthright: "He ate and drank and got up and went and despised his birthright" (my translation of the Hebrew). That is what so many of us do, except we don't do it in one sitting. We do it over a period of years.

You might say (as I used to when defending my unhealthy eating), "I just read about a marathon runner, thin and fit, apparently the picture of health, and he dropped dead of a heart attack. And I just read about a jazz musician who turned one hundred the other day, and he smokes cigars and eats burgers and fries. You just never know why these things happen."

But what we do know is this: the biblical principle of sowing and reaping is true, and if we sow to health, as a rule we will reap health. And if we sow to heart disease and other deadly ailments, as a rule we will reap sickness, disease, and premature death.

If you doubt me, try it out for six months. Get some blood tests done, check your blood pressure, and weigh yourself, then eat a totally healthy diet for the next six months and get checked out again. (For eating recommendations, see chapter 15). Not only will you see a great change on the scale, but you'll see a real difference in your blood levels and blood pressure, along with a real difference in how you feel. Simply stated, bad eating produces bad results, especially over a period of time, while good eating produces good results, especially over a period of time.

Another excuse I used was this: "One generation ago, we were told that certain foods were healthy, and today we're told other foods are healthy and the old 'healthy' ones are not healthy. Everybody's got an opinion, and you have all these competing diet plans. Who knows what's right? Plus I'm in good health overall and I work out heavily, so I must be in good shape."

Yes, it's true that there are competing diet plans—what I advocate is not a diet but a lifestyle change—and yes, it's true that in the past there were different dietary recommendations. But what is undeniable is this: thousands of studies indicate that some foods are healthy and some foods are not, and our bodies are the proof that those studies are right. You could call my old mind-set one of willful ignorance. Perhaps you currently think the way I used to think.

Let's go back to Esau and think in terms of risk and reward. Hebrews urges us not to be like "Esau, who for one morsel of food sold his birthright. For you know that afterward, when he wanted to inherit the blessing, he was rejected. For he found no place for repentance, though he sought it diligently with tears" (Heb. 12:16–17, MEV). For the rest of his life, Esau regretted his decision. It wasn't worth it!

And that's the way it always is with sin. As the old saying goes, sin will take you farther than you planned to go, it will keep you longer than you planned to stay, and it will cost you more than you planned to pay. It's the same with unhealthy eating: the risk is not worth the reward, and sometimes, just as with other choices we make, it is the long-term effect of wrong, small choices that can bring destruction.

As the Puritan Thomas Brooks wrote,

> *... there is great danger, yea, many times most danger in the smallest sins....* Greater sins do sooner startle the soul, and awaken and rouse up the soul to repentance, than less sins do. Little sins often slide into the soul, and breed and work secretly and undiscernibly in the soul, till they come to be so strong, as to trample upon the soul, and to cut the throat of the soul. There is oftentimes greatest danger to our bodies in the least diseases that hang upon us, because we are apt to make light of them, and to neglect the timely use of means for removing them, till they are grown so strong, that they prove mortal to us.[1]

Turning again to the Scriptures, I want to draw your attention to a truth that has burned in my heart for more than thirty years. I have preached about it around the world, and it has never failed to make a deep and lasting impact on the hearers. In fact, I honestly believe that this one, simple truth can change your life forever. It is based on one Hebrew word, and that word is *'acharît* (pronounced ah-kha-REET).[2] Clear your throat and repeat after me: ah-kha-REET. That's it! Say it again slowly: ah-kha-REET.

"But how can one Hebrew word change my life?" you ask. Stay with me and you'll find out.

In the Hebrew language, just as in Arabic, Aramaic, and

the other Semitic languages, many prepositions or words having to do with direction or orientation are derived from parts of the body. For example, in Hebrew the words for "first" or "beginning" come from the word for "head," since in the human body it is the head that comes first. And just as we can speak about being at the "head of the class" in English, so also in Hebrew you can speak about being at the "head" ("top") of the mountain.

Now, the word *'acharît* is related to the Hebrew word for "back," and it literally means "that which comes after; after-effects; final consequences; end."[3] The principle is simple: From our normal vantage point, we cannot see someone's back. We don't see what comes after. And so, if I tore the back of my suit jacket, leaving an ugly hole, you would never know it if you saw me only from the front. From that angle I would look fine. But as soon as I walked past you, you would gasp. Moments ago everything seemed great; from behind it was embarrassing. When you saw my back, the whole picture changed. Instead of looking sharp, I looked sloppy. And that's the biblical principle: from our ordinary, human vantage point we cannot see that which comes after, the final consequences of a matter, the *'acharît*.

But God always sees the whole picture. In His eyes the *'acharît* is always in full view.[4] And if we are to live holy and whole lives, it is crucial that we gain His perspective. In a moment this will all become clear.

KEEP YOUR EYES ON THE *'ACHARÎT*

This word *'acharît* occurs sixty-five times in the Old Testament, but thirteen of those times—i.e., 20 percent of the time—it is found in the book of Proverbs. There is a lesson here! In fact, the whole purpose of Proverbs can be summed up in one verse, Proverbs 19:20: "Listen to counsel and receive discipline/instruction so that you will be wise in your final end" (literally, "in your *'acharit*").[5] That's what really counts. When all is said and done, you will have acted and lived wisely. Your *'acharit* will be blessed.

The problem is that Satan never shows us the *'acharit*. Instead, his whole focus is on the here and now, on the pleasure of the moment, on the need of the hour. And so he does his best to get our eyes off the *'acharit*, the "end" of the story, and that's exactly what happened to Esau. If he had the least bit of foresight, the least bit of measuring the pleasure of the moment with the loss of his birthright, he never would have eaten that stew.

Why then do we often make such foolish life choices? It's because sin is very seductive and because we fail to consider the *'acharit*.

From Nancy: This is such a big issue for so many because when temptation comes, we're always caught up in "the moment" and are completely dulled to the reality of the end. We're unable to see and relate to the regret we're going to feel after we've had our fill. We're numb to the potential destruction that's right around the corner. If we can learn how to focus on the *'acharit* and tune ourselves in to that reality, it can go a long way in helping prevent us from jumping off the cliff. Those few moments of pleasure are not worth the lasting pain.

Let's take a look at a passage in Proverbs 5, one of many in that book warning about the dangers of sexual immorality:

> My son, attend to my wisdom, and bow your ear to my understanding, that you may regard discretion, and that your lips may keep knowledge. For the lips of an immoral woman drip as a honeycomb, and her mouth is smoother than oil. But her end

is bitter as wormwood [literally, her *'acharit* is bitter as wormwood], sharp as a two-edged sword. Her feet go down to death, her steps take hold of Sheol. She does not ponder the path of life; her ways are unstable, and she does not know it.

—PROVERBS 5:1–6, MEV

No matter how good the seductive woman looks, the final consequences of associating with her will be disastrous. Totally.

I read a story in a New York newspaper more than three decades ago that had my stomach in knots for almost two days. A wealthy businessman had been kidnapped. According to the gruesome story, he met an attractive young woman who offered him sex, making arrangements with him to meet her at a specific location another day. But when he met her and went inside the house, he was ambushed by several other men and women, then bound and gagged and brought to an abandoned apartment building in the city. There he was held captive in a room that had been specially prepared for this moment, with extra boards over the windows to muffle the noise of his cries.

What the newspaper then described remained vivid in my mind for many years: They began to torture and abuse this man, burning him with cigarettes over his whole body and sodomizing him with such force that some of his internal organs were severely damaged. They made him relieve himself in a diaper, and for the last five days of his life they starved him as well. And even though his wife agreed to pay a ransom for him, they beat him to death before the money could arrive. My stomach is in knots again even as I write!

If only he could have seen his *'acharit*! If only he could have seen himself screaming in agony, pleading for mercy, tortured and molested, beaten and humiliated, starved and bound—then lying motionless, a bloody corpse. If he only could have seen the final consequences of his adulterous lust, he would have never gone near that young woman, no matter how good-looking she was and no matter what physical pleasures she offered him. He would have sworn off sex for the rest of his life rather than meet such a terrible fate. But he didn't see his *'acharit*!

That's why the warnings in Proverbs are so urgent. There is no hyperbole here!

> Hear me now therefore, O children, and do not depart from the words of my mouth. Remove your way far from her, and do not go near the door of her house, lest you give your honor to others, and your years to the cruel; lest strangers be filled with your wealth, and your labors go to the house of a stranger; and you mourn [the NJPSV has "roar"] at the last [literally, in your *'acharit*!], when your flesh and your body are consumed, and say, "How I have hated instruction, and my heart despised reproof! And I have not obeyed the voice of my teachers, nor inclined my ear to those who instructed me! I was almost in utter ruin in the midst of the congregation and assembly."
>
> —PROVERBS 5:7–14, MEV

I have sat with friends of mine who destroyed their ministries through adultery, their faces twisted with shame, tears of sorrow streaming down their cheeks, their consciences racked with despair and disbelief. And I have prayed silently as I wept with them, "God, don't let me ever forget the expression on his face! Don't let me forget that look of anguish and pain! Let that vivid image stay with me for life." It's not worth it; it's not worth it; it's not worth it! No amount of sexual satisfaction, no amount of romantic excitement, no amount of fulfillment and release is worth forfeiting the ministry. Remember the *'acharit*!

May I ask you, in all candor, if we can draw a real and true parallel when it comes to food? Can I urge you to consider the *'acharit* when it comes to unhealthy eating? Could it be that in your life that double bacon cheeseburger with bottomless fries is no different than that seductive woman? It looks so good; it's so satisfying; you just have to have it—but then it comes back to bite you in the end. Short-term pleasure, long-term pain. Short-term satisfaction, long-term sorrow. The upside is small and fleeting; the downside is large and lasting.

When I used to eat unhealthy foods every day, I would always look forward to dinner, my biggest meal (and often my only real meal) of the day. "What kind of pizza will I get tonight? Maybe some pasta? Perhaps I'll go to a special burger place where they have those great fries. I can hardly wait!" Then once the food was ready, I'd sit there reading a book while I ate or checking e-mails on my cell phone or perusing articles online, hardly even concentrating on the meal, and before I knew it, I was done. Ten, maybe fifteen, maybe twenty minutes, and it was gone.

I would say to myself, "You didn't even concentrate on the food. In a matter of minutes you're done eating, and now you have to wear the results of that food the rest of the day. Why not eat something healthy instead?" It made sense, but I wasn't ready to make the change.

As I was writing some of this very chapter while sitting at the Dallas airport between flights, I saw a man eating a giant burger with fries. He was a pretty big guy, but he had to grasp that burger with two hands, straining to get his mouth around that greasy, fat-filled, unhealthy meal. And what will his reward be if he eats like that on a regular basis? Wads of health-robbing fat; lack of energy; mental dullness; a greater risk of heart disease, stroke, and cancer; and quite possibly a shortened lifespan that robs his family of precious time with him.

Later that same day, while on my flight home, dinner was served, but I declined any food, having had a healthy salad a few hours before and having brought some raw almonds and a healthy snack along for the flight. The man next to me was enjoying a juicy chicken and rice dinner, but the chicken appeared to be loaded with unhealthy extras, and the two rolls he was eating (including my old favorite, the pretzel roll) were dripping in butter.

Did that chicken look good? Did those rolls look appetizing? You bet they did. But I've been there and done that (or, more precisely, eaten that), and as I said in an earlier chapter, my plan was not working. I'm thrilled to be enjoying the benefits of healthy eating and not feeling in the least bit deprived or sorry for myself. To the contrary, I felt sorry for that guy devouring that burger.

I would encourage you to look at unhealthy foods the way you'd look at pornography (or something else that has visual appeal and promises instant gratification but is off limits and destructive). It's not worth it—unless you think that freely eating the unhealthy foods of your choice is worth cutting your days short; suffering terrible, painful disease; reducing your quality of life; and robbing your family and friends of enjoyable years together with you.

The cigarette smoker dying of lung cancer tells us it's not worth it. The alcoholic dying of cirrhosis of the liver tells us it's not worth it. The eighteen-year-old girl with a lifelong STD tells us it's not worth it. And millions of sick (or dead) Americans tell us that unhealthy eating is not worth it. I urge you to consider the *'acharit*!

The same moment I was watching that gentleman wolf down that burger at the airport, I was talking to Nancy on the phone, and she had just listened to comments from a medical doctor who was responding to the idea that it was "extreme" to eat in a totally healthy way. He responded (and

I paraphrase), "What's extreme is cracking open someone's chest and performing a completely preventable quadruple bypass procedure. That's extreme."

He was absolutely right! We must remember the *'acharit*.

The problem is that all too often, we don't see the negative results of our unhealthy eating for decades, and so it might not be until we're in our forties or fifties that our bad habits start to catch up to us. But catch up to us they will, and that's the ultimate principle of the *'acharit*. Look ahead to the final consequences before you satisfy your momentary lust, and you will never give in again. Remember the *'acharit*!

(The day I after I wrote this chapter, I received a phone call from the man who was my best friend during my teenage years. He wanted me to know that a mutual friend of ours, whom I had known since first grade, had just died. When he was just a little boy, he already weighed more than 100 pounds. At the time of his death, suffering from anemia, diabetes, sleep apnea, and COPD [chronic obstructive pulmonary disease], he weighed 375 pounds. He was just sixty years old, like my old best friend and me. So sad and so sobering.)

QUESTIONS FOR REFLECTION

1. In what ways have you been like Esau when it comes to food?

2. What food choices do you make that satisfy for the short term but are destructive for the long term?

3. As you look at your life, what is the *'acharit* for your unhealthy eating?

4. What would be the *'acharit* for a lifestyle transformation of healthy eating?

CHAPTER 13

EXCUSES ARE
FOR WIMPS

A FEW YEARS AGO, I was working out with a couple of my friends, and our trainer was talking about the importance of proper diet along with exercise. Without him accusing any of us or asking for a response, I began to explain how challenging it was for me to eat in an intentionally healthy way, and to tell you the truth, my reasons sounded very convincing—at least to me!

After all, I was constantly on the road, and it seemed that everyone agreed that it was difficult (if not impossible) to maintain a healthy diet while traveling. Plus even when home my schedule was very intense and often erratic. Who had time to plan out each meal or take the time to prepare food at home when it took only a few minutes to grab something to eat on the road? Added to this was the fact that I was often speaking, which meant I had to eat after I spoke at night (which is obviously not the best thing to do) since I could not have a big meal before speaking. And then, my really compelling reason: I liked only a few different foods, and over the years I had added very few (if any) new items to my diet. How could I be expected to eat things I had avoided my entire life?

Our trainer just smiled and listened, we finished our workout, and life went on as usual. Case closed. What else was there to say?

A few days later we were joined in our workout by one of our ministry school grads. He was a little overweight, and as we talked about diet, he began to explain how difficult it was to maintain a healthy lifestyle these days. Both he and his wife worked full time, there was often little time to prepare a meal before they had to go back out to a church meeting or ministry activity, and it was much easier just to eat something quick and unhealthy.

As I listened to him speak, I said to myself, "What wimpy excuses! If he wants to eat better, he can." At that very same moment I said to myself, "And that's how your excuses must sound to others too!"

Really now, isn't it the truth? Our excuses for not getting the job done, showing up late, disappointing someone, or falling short seem so compelling *to us*. But when we hear the same excuses on other people's lips, they sound so lame. That's probably how our excuses sound to them!

The bottom line is that, with God's help, if we really want to make a change or get something done, we can. And the first key to success is to quit blaming others, quit making excuses, take full responsibility for our present situation, and determine—again, with the help of God—to move forward. Cannot our God give us the grace we need to change?

From Nancy: He sure can, and He will, if given the opportunity.

I'm not saying radical change is easy. Obviously it's not; otherwise every one of us would make radical, positive changes all the time. What I'm saying is that I understand the struggle—at least to the extent I struggled for decades to master my diet; others certainly have it much worse—and I was the poster boy for good excuses. That means—to repeat a constant theme of this book—if Nancy and I can make a total lifestyle transformation, anyone can.

The essential foods for life and health that I now eat virtually every day go by the acronym of GBOMBS: Greens, Beans, Onions, Mushrooms, Berries, Seeds (coined by Dr. Fuhrman). Of these, in the past I enjoyed eating some greens (really only lettuce and a little spinach), I detested beans and avoided them at all costs, I loved onions, I would not touch mushrooms, I never ate berries, and as far as seeds were concerned (like raw, unsalted pumpkin and sunflower seeds), they were tolerable, but why eat them?

This was going to be my new diet? And how, pray tell, was I going to get the healthy foods I needed while traveling forty hours to India, let alone once I was *in* India? And what was I going to do when the only meals I could get were at airports?

I started my new lifestyle on August 24, 2014. Over the next four months I traveled to Iowa; California; Missouri; Singapore; California; Texas; Chicago; Hungary; New York; South Carolina; Washington, DC; India; and Malaysia— and note carefully the four international trips in the midst of this schedule. For the Singapore trip, which came very early after my diet change, I was away for almost two weeks, and I had to pay $250 for excess baggage because I needed an extra piece of luggage for all the food Nancy prepared, much of it frozen and packed specially to make it for thirty hours until I arrived at my hotel.

My assistant had to send special instructions ahead on each trip, and sometimes, as in Singapore, I stayed at several different hotels on the same trip, presenting a new set of challenges to add to the mix. But as the old saying goes, where there's a will, there's a way, and for more than two years now I've managed to work things out wherever I was.

From Nancy: This may sound extreme to have to travel with all your food, and it's certainly not necessary for everyone. But because of Mike's complete ignorance of healthy nutritional principles and because of our deal (that I would be the one dictating exactly what he ate), I had the responsibility to make sure he was covered while out of town and out of the country. It was a lot of work, and Mike did his share of complaining about bringing extra luggage, etc., but over time we had fun with it, and now it's just part of our normal routine. We have also been able to pare down considerably, and he even packs for himself now. Thankfully, all his hosts have been extremely accommodating and know exactly what to stock in his hotel refrigerator (and they're always curious and ask about his healthy eating style, admitting that they too need to change their habits).

Sometimes I've had to do without for a meal or two, but it's not the end of the world, and as you can see, I didn't die. (If you're a diabetic or have other health issues, I do understand that sometimes you can't afford to skip a meal. Once again, I remind all of you reading that I'm not giving medical advice; I'm simply sharing my own story.) Sometimes there was a communication mix-up, and when I arrived at the hotel my hosts had the typical gift basket waiting for me in the room, filled with all the goodies I used to eat before. I either gave them back to the hosts, left them for the people cleaning the room, or got rid of them another way. (This has happened quite a few times.)

Often, especially in hotels overseas, there's an assortment of snacks you can purchase, along with free snacks left in the room, and more times than not there are some chocolate delicacies available. The word for this is *temptation*, and temptation is to be resisted. It's no different than having a TV in the room with all kinds of filthy programming available. As a child of God I don't watch the trash, and as a child of God I don't eat the trash. (Speaking for myself, these bad foods are trash to be avoided.)

How about trying to find a healthy meal at an airport, especially in smaller cities where the choices are more limited? Do you know how easy it is to feel deprived as, everywhere you look, people are eating all kinds of enjoyable but unhealthy foods? I once took a picture of an airport sign saying something like, "Healthy Eating Choices," and what followed was a list of very unhealthy food options, including Dunkin' Donuts.

At this point I'm quite used to the fact that, for the most part, I don't eat what other people eat, and when I see one obese person after another trudging past me in the terminals, my heart goes out to them and I'm filled with gratitude for my own radical transformation. And when I see thin people eating a big ice cream cone or downing a slice of pizza dripping with cheese, I simply say to myself, "It didn't work for me!" Plus, who knows what their blood vessels look like? You can be thin and yet unhealthy, and regardless of how you fare at the moment, what you sow today in terms of food, you will reap tomorrow in terms of health.

The bottom line is that *we all have excuses*, and you can see that mine were pretty substantial, at least to me. But once I came to the point of "enough is enough," once I really cried out to the Lord, once I knew that I could not and would not continue going in the direction I was going, I was able to make a total and complete change. I am so thrilled that I did!

ADOPT A NO-EXCUSES MIND-SET

The next time you're reading through the Gospels, take note of how Jesus dealt with excuses. (See, for example, Luke 9:57–62.) The same Savior who was so incredibly merciful and compassionate, the same Lord who would lay down His life for us, His sheep, that same Jesus did not tolerate excuses. He cut through them with surgical precision and exposed what was really behind those excuses: lack of commitment and lack of will.

It's better to say to the Lord, "I confess that I am not willing to change. I admit that I love my food more than I love my health—or even my family. I acknowledge that I'm a slave to bad eating habits. And I'm asking for Your help because I really want to change." He gives grace to the humble, but He resists the proud (Jacob [James] 4:6),[1] and sometimes it is pride that lies at the root of our excuses. We don't like to admit we're wrong.

I was once reading a book written by a friend of mine who had asked for my endorsement. In the book he related that army cadets at West Point had only four options when responding to a commanding officer:

- "Yes, sir."

- "No, sir."

- "I don't understand, sir."

- "No excuses, sir."

After reading that—I never checked the accuracy of the statement, but it did stick with me—I took notice of my tendency to shift the blame for my failures, even in the smallest things. There was always an explanation! Since then, although I haven't been entirely consistent, I've often reminded myself of the "no excuses" mentality, and it really does make a difference in the way you think and the way you live.

How about making a fresh determination today that no matter where you find yourself in life, you'll adopt this "no excuses" mind-set? How about saying, "If I'm overweight or if I'm a slave to bad eating habits, it's no one's fault but my own. No matter what people have done to me, no matter what trauma I've passed through, no matter how hard my life has been—I'm responsible for what goes in my mouth." Will you take ownership of your weight?

Some would say, "But it takes too much time to prepare a healthy meal, and I simply don't have that time." Perhaps you're very busy (most of us can relate), but clock yourself over the course of the day and you'll probably be amazed to see how much time you waste or how much discretionary time you really have. And if, God forbid, your child's health was dependent on you preparing healthy meals for him or her, wouldn't you find the time to do it? Is your own health any less important?

As for taking time, it is true that it takes longer for me to make a smoothie in the morning than to eat a protein bar, but over the course of the day I can eat an apple or some berries as easily as I can eat some pretzels. Plus, if I do invest an extra fifteen minutes in that nutrient-packed smoothie in the morning, I have more energy throughout the day, more than regaining the lost time.

Some would say, "But it costs too much to eat healthy food all the time." Actually, the amount you will save on doctor's bills and other health-related expenses pales in comparison to the amount you will spend on healthy food. And, the truth be told, if you used to eat out a lot (as I did), you'll actually see your food bills drop, as has happened with Nancy and me.

Without a doubt, it can be challenging to prepare healthy meals for yourself and have to cook something else for the rest of the family if they're not eating what you are eating. I haven't had to do this myself, but I know moms who have, and it's not easy for sure. But if your life depended on it—which, in a real sense, it does—you could do it. And perhaps one day the whole family will eat healthily too. After all, if you have younger children, it's not that hard to change their lifestyle.

But can I be really candid for a moment? I have noticed that those people who give me all their food excuses actually refuse to make the choices they can easily make, like portion control, getting rid of bad foods, and adding healthy foods. In other words, let's say you really don't have the money to buy fresh organic veggies and fruits, and let's say you really don't have the time to make healthy salads and meals. What's stopping you from reducing your daily calorie intake? That takes no time, and it certainly saves some money. What's stopping you from skipping that bowl of ice cream after dinner or limiting your intake of potato chips at night or substituting a cucumber for a candy bar?

When you go to a fast-food restaurant, what's stopping you from getting a salad rather than a burger or from getting small fries rather than large fries—or better yet, sliced apples rather than fries? (Remember, when you say, "Supersize my order," you're really saying, "Supersize me!") I am *not* recommending this as a healthy lifestyle change, since it hardly addresses the larger problems (see chapter 15 for more on nutritional tips), but I *am* recommending this as a way to expose excuses. Don't tell me you can't eat less, cut out the worst foods in your diet, cook things in a healthier way, or make daily choices to turn away from gluttony and/or bad eating habits—unless you are completely bound, in which case you acknowledge that before the Lord and humbly ask for His help.

From Nancy: When Mike was still eating poorly, I was the only one in the household eating healthfully, and I had to prepare my own food and eat differently than the rest of the family. Thankfully Mike agreed to eat out more or prepare his own foods. That helped a lot. But there were holidays and family gatherings and special occasions where everyone ate the "usual," and I didn't join in. There were times when I had to excuse myself (remember, sometimes you have to flee!) as well as times when I was strong enough to sit with everyone while they ate pizza and I didn't. The question was, how badly did I want it? It feels like such a challenge in the beginning, but the rewards far outweigh the sacrifices.

Nancy and I were once talking to a friend of ours who suffered from type 2 diabetes, and she said to him, "You know your condition is completely reversible if you'll switch to a vegan diet."[2] He replied, "I know, but I hate veggies." At least he was being honest, but at what cost?

I propose to you that you get on the scale after reading this chapter (unless you're too heavy for a conventional scale; in that case, just look in the mirror), face the facts squarely, and say to the Lord, "No excuses, Sir!" And if you recently got a bad medical report that could largely be reversed through healthy eating and exercise, hold that report in your hand and say to the Lord, "No excuses, Sir!"

I know it's easier to take a blood pressure pill than to change your lifestyle, but that pill doesn't truly address the root problem and, even more seriously, that pill could do serious damage to your liver or other organs. The same holds true for medicine designed to reduce your cholesterol levels: the medicine masks the symptoms rather than corrects the problem, also creating new potential problems of their own. It is far better to reverse the symptoms by addressing the cause, enabling you to get off the medication entirely and greatly improve your health.

Unfortunately, most doctors in America don't focus on nutritional remedies, thereby enabling us to continue our unhealthy lifestyles: "The doctor told me I need to take these pills because my blood pressure is high," rather than, "The doctor told me that I'm 100 pounds overweight, that I'm running the risk of greatly shortening my life as well as reducing the quality of my life in the years I have remaining, and he urged me to make radical changes to my diet." In the first case, our excuses win the day ("I'm not obese because of bad choices I make; I'm just a heavy person."); in the second case, we have to take responsibility for our condition ("I'm obese because of the bad choices I make.")

I remember a conversation my father once had with a psychiatrist about smoking cigarettes. I was a new believer at the time, so I was probably about seventeen or eighteen. My dad was close to sixty, and he had been smoking since he was a little boy. He asked the doctor, "Is there some kind of hypnosis you can perform on me to help me stop smoking?"

To my shock, the doctor replied to my dad (a man I deeply respected), "What are you, some kind of baby? If you want to stop smoking, stop."

That was like a slap in the face to my dear father, but he quit smoking shortly after that without any outside help or intervention.

I'm not saying everyone can do what he did, and trust me, I do understand the power of addictions, especially food addictions. I'm simply urging you to stop making excuses, to stop avoiding reality, to stop blaming others, and to take responsibility for where you find yourself. Once you do that, you can work on making the changes necessary to achieve vibrant health—at least to the extent your health depends on your diet.

From Nancy: For my part, I never really made excuses in the sense that Mike is talking about in this chapter. Whining about having to shop more or cook more or feeling left out at family gatherings was not actually anything that would prevent me from changing. Those were just nuisances to complain about. I knew had to do something. I knew I had to change. I just wasn't in the mood to do it today. Tomorrow I'll do it.

QUESTIONS FOR REFLECTION

1. What are some strategies to overcome your biggest reasons for not beginning a healthier lifestyle?

2. What have been your main excuses in the past for not changing your eating habits?

3. How do you view the excuses that others make to you for their failings?

4. Are you willing to say to the Lord right now, "No excuses, Sir!"?

CHAPTER 14

HOLINESS PRINCIPLES FOR WHOLESOME EATING

L ET'S GO BACK to the Garden of Eden. *The very first temptation Satan presented to the human race was a food temptation.* I've read the story for more than four decades, and I could quote it back to you from memory, but it was only recently that I recognized how much *food itself* played an important role in the temptation.

From Nancy: Think of the crowds that came flocking to Jesus after He multiplied the fishes and the loaves. He said to them, "Truly, truly, I say to you, you are seeking me, not because you saw signs, but because you ate your fill of the loaves" (John 6:26). This is really incredible. Here is Jesus healing the sick, opening blind eyes, setting captives free, and working all kinds of miracles, but the crowds weren't coming because of that. They were coming for the food!

Let's revisit the account in Genesis 3:1–6, where the serpent tempts Eve to sin. The text states, "Now the serpent was more crafty than any other beast of the field that the LORD God had made" (Gen. 3:1). Satan is not mentioned by name here, but he's obviously the one working through the serpent.

"He said to the woman, 'Did God actually say, "You shall not eat of any tree in the garden"?'" (Gen. 3:1). In keeping with his diabolical nature, he actually twists the Word of the Lord, thereby making God look suspect.

Eve is quick to correct him, but while doing so, she adds to what God had previously spoken to Adam. "And the woman said to the serpent, 'We may eat of the fruit of the trees in the garden'"—so far, so good—"'but God said, "You shall not eat of the fruit of the tree that is in the midst of the garden, neither shall you touch it, lest you die"'"+ (Gen. 3:2–3). That's exactly true, except Eve added in, "neither shall you touch it." So already we see the very human tendency of adding to God's commands. This is a very dangerous practice.

"But the serpent said to the woman, 'You will not surely die. For God knows that when you eat of it your eyes will be opened, and you will be like God, knowing good and evil'" (Gen. 3:4–5). He was lying! On the one hand, he knew that Adam's and Eve's eyes would be opened when they ate of the tree, but he also knew they would lose the childlike innocence they had. (Can you imagine being perfectly developed, fully mature adults but with the innocence of a little baby?)

Why didn't Eve resist the serpent? Why didn't she say, "I will not listen to you! You're challenging me to question my Creator"? Let's see what the Scripture says. I'll emphasize two key phrases we may have overlooked in the past: "So when the woman saw that the tree was *good for food*, and that it was a *delight to the eyes*, and that the tree was to be desired to make one wise, she took of its fruit and ate, and she also gave some to her husband who was with her, and he ate" (Gen. 3:6, emphasis added).

And that is what we call the fall of man. It began with a food temptation!

Eve was tempted to disobey God not just by the lure of becoming like God and knowing good and evil. She was tempted first by the lust of the flesh for food—the fruit of the tree was good for food—and by the lust of the eyes—the fruit of the tree looked really good—as well as by the desire to become wise. That's why she took and ate and gave some to her husband, who also ate willfully. (It's important to note that while Eve may have been deceived into sin, Adam outright rebelled.)

Now take a look in 1 John 2:15–17, where John makes this striking statement: "Do not love the world or the things in the world. If anyone loves the world, the love of the Father is not in him. For all that is in the world—*the lust of the flesh, the lust of the eyes, and the pride of life*—is not of the Father, but is of the world. The world and its desires are passing away, but the one who does the will of God lives forever" (MEV, emphasis added).

This is a recap of the temptation in the garden: the lust of the flesh (the fruit was good for food), the lust of the eyes (the fruit looked really good), and the pride of life (the fruit would make you wise). This is the destructive spirit of the world, and it is antithetical to the love of the Father, by which I mean that living for these lusts and finding the meaning of one's life in these lusts is antithetical to leading a life filled with God.

This doesn't mean that we can't enjoy a tasty meal, that the food we eat needs to look like garbage, or that we can't have nice things in life. It means that being driven, dominated, and controlled by these fleshly lusts is of the world, not the

Father. And it means that the lust for food can be every bit as destructive as the lust for sex, money, or power.

For some of you reading this book, the lust for food is the number one lustful desire you wrestle with and the one that cripples you the most. The good news is that the same holiness principles that will help you overcome these other lusts will help you overcome the lust for food.

All of us are familiar with the racy ads that constantly appear on TV, most often featuring attractive women who appeal to male lusts. Why else are half-naked, alluringly posed women appearing in car or hamburger ads? They are there simply to get more eyes on the product being advertised, even though they have no connection to the product itself. The ads are just plain seductive. (Good-looking men are now being used to attract female—or gay—buyers these days.)

Well, for the most part food ads don't rely on the presence of beautiful women (putting some notorious burger ads aside); they rely on the seductive images of the foods themselves. How we drool over those images! Just think about some of your favorite meals, then think of the ads that promote your favorite restaurants. It's the food equivalent of porn. How sumptuous and delicious and appealing—and deadly!

For me, as a pizza devotee of more than forty years, those pizza commercials could really appeal to me. That thick cheese dripping off the slice seemed ready to drip into my mouth. There's even cheese in the crust now, which is bathed in garlic too. And those cheese bread appetizers to start things off, dipped in marinara sauce, seemed to call to me.

Not anymore! I can look at it and say, "That looks absolutely delicious, but it's not for me. I'm free." How wonderful indeed it feels to be free.

Almost twenty years ago I wrote an entire book on holiness titled *Go and Sin No More* (yes, that's pretty direct, but I got the words from Jesus Himself; see John 8:11). Some of the principles I articulated in that book can be of help to you in your battle against food lusts. Let me share some of them here with you. They overlap with some of the other chapters laid out in this book, so what's written here will reinforce and sharpen what you've read so far.

CUT IT OUT, DON'T CUT IT BACK

Listen to what Jesus said about dealing with sinful tendencies in our lives:

> Woe to the world because of temptations! For it must be that temptations come, but woe to that man by whom the temptation comes! Therefore if your hand or your foot causes you to sin, cut it off and throw it away. It is better for you to enter life lame or maimed than having two hands or two feet to be thrown into eternal fire. And if your eye causes you to sin, pluck it out and throw it away. It is better for you to enter life with one eye than having two eyes to be thrown into the fire of hell.
>
> —MATTHEW 18:7–9, MEV

From Nancy: How can you argue with the words of Jesus? What we have to do is pretty simple and straightforward.

New Testament scholar D. A. Carson explains the significance of these words:

> Cutting off or gouging out the offending part is a way of saying that Jesus' disciples must deal radically with sin. Imagination is a God-given gift; but if it is fed dirt by the eye, it will be dirty. All sin, not least sexual sin, begins with the imagination. Therefore what feeds the imagination is of

maximum importance in the pursuit of kingdom righteousness....Not everyone reacts the same way to all objects. But if...your eye is causing you to sin, gouge it out; or at very least, don't look....The alternative is sin and hell, sin's reward. The point is so fundamental that Jesus doubtless repeated it on numerous occasions.[1]

There are few things more radical than amputation. Doctors cut off hands, feet, and legs only as a last resort. They do it because they have no choice. If they don't, the infection will spread, destroying the whole body. So it's either one limb that goes or the whole body that dies. And once the amputation is done, it can't be undone. Once the limb is severed it will never be used again. Yet Jesus tells us to amputate our hands or feet if they cause us to sin.

Of course, this is *spiritual* imagery that graphically explains the ruthless way in which we must deal with sinful tendencies and habits, so you can put the meat cleaver or hatchet away for now! But let's not weaken the force of Jesus's words. They are absolutely radical, totally extreme, completely final: "Cut off that hand and throw it away"—even if it's your right hand, the hand that you rely on in your daily labor, the hand with which you write, your strong hand. Even that hand must go if it leads you into sin.

The same goes for our eyes. He said that if our eye—even our right eye—causes us to sin, we should gouge it out and throw it away. Think of it! Military men in hand-to-hand combat gouge out the enemy soldier's eye only when there is no other way to subdue or stop him. Even if he survives, he's blind for life. But Jesus said it's better for people to be right with God—even if it means being blind or maimed—than to have two hands, two feet, and two eyes and go straight to hell, "where their worm does not die and the fire is not quenched" (Mark 9:48). And notice that Jesus spoke about three parts of the body: our hands, signifying what we do; our feet, signifying where we go; and our eyes, signifying what we see and desire.

The lesson here is simple. If you know certain foods are wrong for you—they're either unhealthy in and of themselves, they're addictive, or they lead you into destructive eating habits—cut them out entirely. Cutting them back rather than cutting them out means that they will keep growing back. (For more on this, see chapter 11, "Blessed with the Gift of Being 'All In.'")

LITTLE FOXES SPOIL THE VINES

As I stated previously, the Puritan leader Thomas Brooks wrote, "*There is great danger, yea, many times most danger, in the smallest sins.*"[2] The concept of "little foxes spoiling the vines" comes from Song of Solomon 2:15, "Catch the foxes for us, the little foxes that spoil the vineyards, for our vineyards are in blossom" (MEV). As Charles Spurgeon commented, "If thou wouldst live with Christ, and walk with Christ, and see Christ, and have fellowship with Christ, take heed of 'the little foxes that spoil the vines, for our vines have tender grapes.'"[3]

How does this apply to food? Many of us focus on the "big" spiritual matters, things like prayer; reading the Word; sharing our faith; spending quality time with our spouses, children, or friends; turning away from sexual sins, drugs, or drunkenness; or standing up for social justice. These are certainly big, without a doubt; some of them are absolutely foundational. But what about the sins involving food? Could it be that for some of us our eating habits are like the little foxes that spoil the vines? Could it be that it is our obesity—which is the result of our food addictions, our unhealthy eating habits, or our lack of discipline—that is hindering our walk with the Lord? (For more on this, see chapter 5, "Too Fat to Fly.")

Think of it like this: if the essence of holiness can be described as loving and serving God with an undivided heart, then anything that divides your heart—even if it is "neutral" in and of itself—is sin. The same can be said for anything that dulls or distracts your heart. It's sin, even if it's commendable in the eyes of man, even if it's clean in the eyes of man, even if it's correct in the eyes of man. If it takes you away from devotion to the Lord or blunts your spiritual sharpness, it's sin for you.

And what if the thing that's blunting your spiritual sharpness is *not* neutral in itself? What if it's actually bad for you? Those late-night snacks could be clogging your arteries. Those decadent desserts could be dulling your brain. Those all-you-can-eat buffets may be cutting your life short. Here too we need to be vigilant. Those gigantic portions at your favorite restaurant could be blunting your prayer life. (How often have you had a wonderful time in prayer after gorging yourself? I certainly haven't.)

Consider it from this angle. We can't watch whatever we want on TV or in the movies. Some things are not suitable for God's children. In the same way, we can't say whatever we want to say or think whatever we want to think or have a romantic relationship with whomever we want to. Of course not. There are guidelines for holy living laid out in the Word, and the Spirit within writes God's laws on our hearts.

Then why do we have a different standard when it comes to food? Who says that we can eat whatever we want to eat? Perhaps some foods are off limits, not in terms of dietary laws, but in terms of the stewardship of our bodies.

Don't let little food foxes spoil your vines!

THERE'S ALWAYS A WAY OF ESCAPE

No matter where you find yourself today, even if you're 400 pounds overweight and your life is collapsing around you, even if you've tried a hundred different diets and you're heavier today than you've ever been, with the Lord there *is* a way of escape. You don't have to live and die in obesity, shame, and bondage. Your life can be transformed, just as Nancy's was and just as mine was. God is no respecter of persons.

Look at this very serious passage in 2 Peter:

> For if God did not spare the angels that sinned, but cast them down to hell and delivered them into chains of darkness to be kept for judgment; and if He did not spare the ancient world, but saved Noah, a preacher of righteousness, with seven others, when He brought a flood upon the world of the ungodly; and if He condemned the cities of Sodom and Gomorrah to destruction by reducing them to ashes, making them an example to those afterward who would live ungodly lives; and if He delivered righteous Lot, who was distressed by the filthy conduct of the wicked (for that righteous man lived among them, and what he saw and heard of their lawless deeds tormented his righteous soul day after day); *then the Lord knows how to rescue the godly from trial,* and to keep the unrighteous under punishment for the Day of Judgment.
>
> —2 PETER 2:4–9, MEV, EMPHASIS ADDED

This applies to food strongholds as well!

When Nancy changed her lifestyle, we both "knew" it couldn't work for me, since 1) I didn't "like" the foods I would need to eat; 2) I would have to give up almost all the foods I really did like; and 3) I was on the road all the time and it was not practical. Well, surprise, surprise, God gave me grace and Nancy gave me practical suggestions, and all of these seemingly insurmountable objections have been left in the dust. The Lord answered our prayers!

Your situation may appear far more hopeless than mine (or Nancy's; her story was different than mine in many ways), but the same Lord can deliver you and give you a plan of attack or make a way of escape or send friends to help or change your desires or do something brilliantly creative and out of the box as only He can do. You need only cry out to Him from the depths of your heart, refusing to quit until He answers and taking whatever steps you're able to take.

From Nancy: You do what you can and He'll do what you can't.

The Lord made a way of escape for me in 1971, setting me free from two years of heavy drug use, including shooting heroin, and He has been making them for me ever since. The fact is, there's always a way of escape for God's people. None of us have to fall beyond the point of recovery, ever. The Word is totally clear: "Cast your cares on the Lord, and he will sustain you; he will never permit the righteous to be moved" (Ps. 55:22)—and *never* means "never," as surely as God is God.

And what if we stagger a little, hit hard by temptation and trial? Even then we have a promise: "The steps of a man are made firm by the Lord; He delights in his way. Though he falls, he will not be hurled down, for the Lord supports him with His hand" (Ps. 37:23–24, mev). We don't have to hit the deck and stay there, no matter how heavily the enemy attacks. If you "put on the full armor of God," then "when the day of evil comes," you can "stand your ground, and after you have done everything," you can stand (Eph. 6:13, niv). You may stumble. You may stagger. But you need never go down for the count.

In light of these assurances—and no doubt, based on personal experience too—Jude could speak of God as the One "who is able to keep you from falling and to present you blameless before the presence of His glory with rejoicing" (Jude 24, MEV). Rather than dreading the day when we will stand before God—as if it would be time of abject terror causing us to hang our heads in great shame—we can look forward to that time with great joy. What glorious keeping power! God can finish what He starts (1 Cor. 1:8; Phil. 1:6; Heb. 12:1), and He can keep and deliver His own. He's been doing it for quite a long time. Still, He will not do it without our active cooperation. He will not force us to flee.

Of course, if we put our confidence in ourselves, trusting in our strength and ability, we might be headed for a crash. Paul warned the Corinthians about this very danger, reminding them of Israel's history: "So, if you think you are standing firm, be careful that you don't fall!" (1 Cor. 10:12, NIV). Complacency and pride are twin sins that will slay any giant, no matter how big and strong. They are fatal to smug saints too! But if our trust is in the faithfulness of the Lord, we can be assured of this: "No temptation has taken you except what is common to man. God is faithful, and He will not permit you to be tempted above what you can endure, but will with the temptation also make a way to escape, that you may be able to bear it" (1 Cor. 10:13, MEV).

Often the way of escape God provides is a simple one: Run for your life! Flee! Don't try to be a hero and be strong and put yourself in the place of temptation day after day, fighting your hardest to resist. Use the wisdom the Lord has given you and get away from that source of temptation. When I stopped doing drugs, I stopped going to parties as well since getting high was one of the main things we did at those parties. In the same way, when Nancy changed her lifestyle, she found it necessary at times to stay away from certain gatherings or to avoid eating out since it was hard to be around all that tempting food without eating. So rather than pray for strength to resist that doughnut at Dunkin' Donuts, avoid going there entirely if you can.

Because I'm always on the road, I found myself at restaurants and on long flights from the earliest days of my new lifestyle, which meant I had to resist temptation all the time. You can't flee from an airplane flying at thirty thousand feet! Bad food was constantly available, from my hotel room to the restaurant to the airport to the flight, but by God's grace I was able to say no all the time. At the same time I asked my hosts to take me to restaurants with salad bars and give me plenty of fruit in my room. The last place I wanted to be was in a terrific Italian restaurant or famous pizzeria. Why play with fire?

There are those times when pressures build up and we find ourselves in a squeeze, feeling "overmatched" for the moment. And even though we have at our disposal the authority of the Word of God, the authority of the name of Jesus, and the authority of the indwelling Spirit, Satan can be very clever, setting up a situation tailor-made for our demise. Suddenly, we find ourselves facing the "perfect" temptation. It relentlessly stares us down and blocks out all thoughts of spiritual authority or victory. We can't remember a single scripture to quote, the very thought of rebuking the devil sounds like a joke, and all our wisdom and maturity seem to have vanished into thin air. What can we do? Pray, "Help me, Lord! Deliver me, God! Please get me out of this mess! Show me the way!" He can! He has! He will!

He will create an escape route if He has to, or He will help us get back to our senses so that "spell" is broken. One way or another, He will make a way even where there is no way. He specializes in supernatural deliverances. After all, He's the Deliverer, and He can deliver you from food addictions, food strongholds, unhealthy eating habits, and obesity. It's time for your deliverance!

QUESTIONS FOR REFLECTION

1. Do you realize that the lust for food can be as deadly as any other kind of lust? Can you see your food desires as dangerous lusts?

2. Is there something in your diet or lifestyle that God is calling you to "cut out" rather than "cut back"?

3. What are the little food foxes that are spoiling your vines?

4. Do you believe that God can give you a way of escape? If not, why not?

CHAPTER 15

TEN RECOMMENDATIONS FOR A HEALTHY LIFESTYLE

A S I STATED in the Preface, I am neither a medical doctor nor a nutritionist (my PhD is in Near Eastern Languages and Literatures), but I can share with you what Nancy and I have learned from others and what we have lived out in our own lives. It was Nancy who first discovered the writings and videos of Dr. Joel Fuhrman, who became well-known for his bestselling book *Eat to Live*, and his materials had a revolutionary impact on her life.

She had studied nutrition for years and tried various eating programs, but nothing seemed to work long term in terms of weight loss, and she knew she wasn't getting everything she needed nutritionally on these different programs. But she didn't know exactly what she was missing, and there were so many opinions out there, it was dizzying. When she read Dr. Fuhrman's books, the light went on for her, and she realized that his material answered the questions she had been asking, and it was backed up by medical science.

You can read Nancy's personal story in appendix A—I think you'll agree with me that her story is the best part of the book!—and we both highly recommend that you get Dr. Fuhrman's more recent book *The End of Dieting*. Our hope is that with the spiritual motivation found in these pages coupled with the practical (and motivational) guidelines Dr. Fuhrman lays out, your life will be radically changed—for the rest of your life.

KEYS TO A NEW WAY OF LIFE

While the ten keys presented in this chapter do not take the place of reading *The End of Dieting* (or any other books you find helpful), they summarize important truths that provide the foundation for your new way of life.

1. Forget about dieting. You need a lifestyle change.

According to a May 4, 2016, e-blast from Dr. Fuhrman, a study published in the journal *Obesity* found that six years after their initial weight loss, thirteen of the fourteen contestants had regained a significant amount of weight, and four were heavier than before they participated in the show *The Biggest Loser*. The study measured both the contestants' weight and their metabolic rate. The reason for this? "The human body adapts to weight loss by slowing calorie expenditure," Dr. Fuhrman explains, "increasing appetite, and promoting fat storage. If you regain the weight, these adaptations will make losing weight the second time more difficult than the first."[1]

So, the struggle you have with what's called yo-yo dieting—losing weight, gaining it back, losing it again, gaining it back again—is not simply the result of lack of willpower on your part. It's also a matter of a nonworkable plan, since if you lose weight the wrong way, your own body makes it harder to keep it off.[2]

That's why Dr. Fuhrman and others recommend a totally new lifestyle and a totally new approach to food, what he calls "the Nutritarian way of eating."[3]

His conclusion? Diets fail because of lack of proper education, meaning people don't understand what a healthy human diet really looks like. So rather than eating in a healthy way that can be maintained for a lifetime, shows like *The Biggest Loser* offer "a formula for failure and disease." This leads naturally to the next point.

2. Don't cut back on the bad foods. Cut the bad foods out, then replace them with good foods.

If you realize that bad foods really are bad for you, then it's best to cut them out entirely rather than just cutting them back. Otherwise it's much easier to fall back into your old, unhealthy eating habits since you're keeping temptation around on a regular basis. Also, when you only cut back on bad foods, you continue to put unhealthy fuel into your system. What's the purpose of that?

Conversely, when you replace the bad food with good food, over time your palate will be retrained, and you'll enjoy the good stuff the way you used to enjoy the bad stuff. But if you keep eating the bad stuff, your taste buds will never change. Plus, when you eat only healthy foods, they quickly take the place of the bad foods, meaning you will no longer crave the unhealthy stuff. Why make life more difficult for yourself by taking in just enough of the bad foods to keep those addictions alive? And that leads to point number 3.

3. Recognize that food addictions are as real as any other addiction, and they are some of the deadliest addictions we can have.

The other day, I saw a humorous meme on Facebook that said, "Donut Fact #18: Donuts are healthier than crystal meth." Maybe so, but not by much!

One of my favorite doughnuts was the Dunkin' Donuts Chocolate Glazed Cake. (Better still was the double chocolate version, where this already rich doughnut had another layer of chocolate on top.) According to the Calorie King website, there are 370 calories in a single doughnut, including 216 from fat, which equals 37 percent of the recommended daily value of fat content and 55 percent of the recommended daily value of saturated fat content.[4] That means that with just two of these doughnuts—not mentioning anything else you eat all day—you have already exceeded the recommended daily allowance of saturated fat content and have reached 74 percent of the recommended daily allowance of total fat. (And we won't even get started on all the harmful chemicals and additives that are packed in those doughnuts.)

Let's say you decided to really splurge and had those doughnuts with a 24-ounce Starbucks Java Chip Frappuccino® Blended Coffee with whole milk and whipped cream. You've just added another 600 calories to your intake for the day (with the two doughnuts, you'd be at 1340 calories; I live on less than 2,000 calories per day), including another 14 grams of saturated fat, representing the total recommended daily allowance.[5] (This means that you would already have consumed more than twice the recommended daily allowance of saturated fat just with your coffee and doughnuts!)

From Nancy: For me, 1,340 calories would just about push me over my daily caloric intake—and that's simply for a little, snacky breakfast food. What about lunch, dinner, and my favorite bedtime snack? That can add up to thousands of additional calories. No wonder we're getting fatter and fatter as the years go by.

Perhaps you say, "So what's the big deal about having all these fats?" The American Heart Association website has your answer: "Eating foods that contain saturated fats raises the level of cholesterol in your blood. High levels of LDL cholesterol in your blood increase your risk of heart disease and stroke."[6] That Frappuccino and those doughnuts *greatly* increase your risk of heart disease and stroke, and that's just one example of unhealthy eating.

For the most part a significant percentage of the typical American diet is unhealthy, and therefore, in ultimate terms, deadly. Added to this is the addictive nature of many of these foods—I shared earlier in the book how it was easier for me to give up drugs than to give up chocolates and other treats—and you really do have a recipe for disaster.[7]

In his book *Breaking the Food Seduction: The Hidden Reasons Behind Food Cravings—and 7 Steps to End Them Naturally*, Dr. Neal Barnard begins by first discussing "The Seductions," explaining physiologically how we become addicted to certain foods. The titles of the chapters that follow say it all: "Sweet Nothings: The Sugar Seduction"; "Give Me Chocolate or Give Me Death: The Chocolate Seduction"; "Opiates on a Cracker: The Cheese Seduction"; and "The Sizzle: The Meat Seduction."[8] When we fail to take these seductions seriously, we fail ourselves. It doesn't mean you're a bad person if you have bad eating habits. It means you need to have serious resolve to make a change. But people make these changes every day, including atheists and nonbelievers who rely totally on willpower. Surely we who have God's help can make a change.

4. Learn the difference between toxic hunger and true hunger.

This is something Dr. Fuhrman stresses and Nancy helped me to realize.[9] In the past Nancy would see me snacking and say, "Didn't you just eat a couple of hours ago?" I'd reply, "But I'm hungry," to which she'd say, "No, you're not." (Remember: we're Jews from New York, so being candid is in our blood.)

Obviously, I wasn't hungry in terms of starving—(Nancy says it would have been very difficult for someone with ninety-five pounds of excess fat to starve after going just a few hours without eating!)—but I really did feel the desire to eat. Some of this was simply the lust for food, but some of it was toxic hunger. As I explained earlier, toxic hunger is what we feel when our body is deprived of toxic, addictive foods and our stomachs growl and we get a headache or the shakes or feel faint or weak. These symptoms are not a sign of hunger (true, normal hunger doesn't bring these symptoms with it), and they will disappear once we break free from the addictions. Once you start eating healthily and you get hungry, you won't get a headache, the shakes, or feel weak. This sounds very foreign to many of us since we're so used to these "signs" of hunger, but they're actually signs of addiction.

When you learn to recognize true hunger, which won't come every couple of hours if you're eating properly, you'll learn to eliminate snacking, which is our next item on the list.

5. Don't snack between meals.

Snacking is often one of the biggest reasons we gain extra weight as well as a real hindrance to weight loss, and that's for a few obvious reasons. First, we're eating when we don't need to eat because our bodies are not truly in need of nutrients, which means we're just adding extra calories for the day. And do any of us eat smaller portions in our meals to make up for adding snacking calories? Most of the times not.

Second, for the most part we're eating foods that are more

harmful than helpful since we tend to snack on the least healthy foods. (In other words, we're much more likely to snack on chips than on broccoli.) Third, we're not eating to get a needed meal into our system but rather we're eating out of boredom, food addiction, anger, pain, reward, frustration, lust for food, or whatever. Don't let snacking be your downfall, and if you have to snack, eat something totally healthy. It's important that we learn to live, thrive, and enjoy life without eating all the time. (Of course, if you have a medical condition that requires that you eat more frequently, this tip will need to be modified.)

6. Recognize that your stomach is not your god and that unhealthy eating might very well be a sin for you.

While these words would not have as much meaning to a nonbeliever, they certainly have meaning to us. We are children of God, redeemed by the blood of Jesus, indwelt by the Spirit, empowered by the Word, and overcomers by our very nature—our new nature in Jesus. Many of us have been set free from drugs, alcohol, gambling, or other life-controlling addictions. Surely we won't let food addictions conquer us. Surely our stomach is not our god!

And once you recognize unhealthy eating to be sinful, just as many other habits and choices and behaviors are sinful, you will be more determined to change your life. When it comes to unhealthy eating, it is potentially sinful because it is so destructive, addictive, draining, and deadly.

7. Identify the main psychological reasons that you overeat (or eat unhealthy foods).

As I mentioned in chapter 9, for me, food was a reward, and once I broke free from my food addictions, I realized that the battle was far from over. I had to reprogram my mind in terms of how I related to food and why I ate. This was really liberating for me, and it was a big key for the long haul. I still enjoy eating, and I look forward to my daily meals. But I don't live to eat; I eat to live.

Some people overeat because they've suffered a deep emotional trauma and eating has been their place of escape and comfort. (Some foods really are "comfort foods" in more ways than one.) Others overeat for different reasons that are equally deep and entrenched in their lives, while still others simply love certain foods and are addicted to them. For those of you whose food struggles relate to deep spiritual or emotional issues, you might need godly counsel to help you get to the root of the problem. At the least, when you begin to envision this radical new way of living, some of these deep fears or powerful strongholds might rise to the surface, in which case you can work with the Lord (which can include a trusted counselor) to address these problems. Jesus can deliver us from these things too.

8. Understand that food is the fuel for your life.

Do you want to run your race so as to win? Do you want to fulfill your life calling? Do you want to finish well and not just start well? Do you want to persevere to the end, not to mention have energy and focus on a daily basis? Then you'll need some good fuel, and that means healthy eating.

Stop and think about it for a moment. You have only one life, but you could cut it short or greatly diminish its potential in other ways by unhealthy eating. Are you willing to sacrifice the quality and quantity of your life to satisfy the lusts of the stomach?

9. Realize that exercise is important, but it's no substitute for a change in your eating habits.

Trust me. I did some *serious* exercising when I was overweight, and I outworked young men who were in pretty good shape. Yet I remained overweight, my cholesterol was too high, and my blood pressure was even higher. And who knows what else was brewing in my body.

Yes, exercise is important, but put first things first and begin by changing your food habits. Then you'll be able to exercise even more, and the exercising will be far more fruitful.

Today, intensive exercising plays an important role in my life. I thrive in it and am blessed in many ways by the benefits of it. But again, first things first. Let exercise go along with your overall lifestyle change and don't think that exercise can take the place of healthy eating.

10. Resolve that today is the day to make a change. Tomorrow never comes.

Consider this: If you don't determine to make a change now, then when? How many more books like this do you need to read? How many stories like Nancy's and mine do you need to hear? How many more pounds do you need to gain or how many new health crises do you need to endure before you say, "Enough is enough!"?

God will give you grace if you humble yourself and ask for His help. He did it for us. He'll do it for you.

We are cheering you on, and the Lord Himself is for you, not against you. Take the plunge today and never look back. It's time to break the stronghold of food! You'll never be the same.

QUESTIONS FOR REFLECTION

1. Which items on this list of keys to a new way of life most resonate with you and why?

2. Which items on this list most trouble you (or intimidate or scare you) and why?

3. Have you tried to exercise your fat away rather than get rid of your fat through healthy eating? How did that work out for you?

4. Are you willing to say to God (and those close to you), "By Your grace, Lord, I'm in, starting today"? If so, what are the first steps you need to take?

NANCY'S STORY

M Y STORY OF overweight (and food addiction) is very different from my husband's. In many ways, I believe his issues with food were child's play in comparison. It was not a cloud over his entire life like it was in mine. Of course, he has own story to tell, recognizing how bound he was by certain foods and also hating to be fat.

There might be some who read his story and cannot relate because of the apparent mildness of what he went through. So throughout the book I've added my experience for those who say to themselves, "He just doesn't understand and truly has no clue what extreme food addiction is." In this appendix you can read my story from beginning to end, all in one place.

I can tell you I understand. For those struggling with it, it's a stronghold beyond all strongholds. It's *the* stronghold in their lives. It permeates everything, controls everything, and affects everything.

Being overweight has dominated so much of my life. I was the typical yo-yo dieter, always dieting and losing weight and gaining whatever I'd lost by returning to my "normal" eating habits. I absolutely despised being overweight and felt terrible all the time. I was exhausted and barely left the house. There was no physical position that was comfortable for me. Whether it was sitting in a chair or lying in bed, my body felt awful. I ached from head to toe and knew I was killing myself with food.

As for my social life, well, I had no life! I barely left the house. I had removed myself from all social functions because I was just too ashamed of the way I looked and felt. I had very little energy to do normal, everyday tasks. My life was on hold. I'm not even sure how much I weighed because I didn't have the courage to get on the scale the day I firmly decided to make a complete lifestyle change. I waited about a week before I actually weighed myself. I was 195.5 pounds, so I'm pretty sure I was close to 200 pounds when I started— and I'm only 5 feet 2 inches!

I usually ate whatever I wanted in enormous quantities, and that certainly didn't include fruits and vegetables. I loved highly processed, fatty, salty foods; pastas; cheeses; cream sauces; and, of course, gooey chocolate desserts. No wonder I felt sick all the time. I needed an absolute, complete lifestyle change, a new way of living and not just some diet fad that would be tossed aside once I reached my goal weight.

In the past, on several occasions I had tried to adjust my diet by attempting to go vegan but never really had all the pertinent information to do this healthfully. I knew I was missing key knowledge. I got to the point where I was feeling so bad that it actually scared me. My cholesterol, glucose, and blood pressure, which were always in normal ranges, were now creeping up (although I didn't pay much attention to this initially).

I knew I had to do something but did not have a clear direction as to how to get the weight off and regain my health. I had decided to start a healthy diet in July 2012, but I knew I needed something different than what I'd tried in the past. I was so discouraged because of my past failures and didn't have the heart to start the same old dieting routine all over again. I desperately searched the Internet for some help and came across Dr. Joel Fuhrman's website and his "nutritarian" way of eating.

My first reaction was, "Well, here's just another dieting gimmick." But the more I looked through the website and researched his information, the more convinced I became that this was not just another gimmick. Everything made so much sense to me. I actually joined Dr. Fuhrman's Member Center, purchased his books *Eat to Live* and *Eat for Health*, and was on my way. I devoured and made use of everything on the website. The articles and teleconferences as well as the discussion forums were invaluable to me, and still are. (I'm not necessarily advocating or pushing that everyone join their online community. I'm just saying that along with the nutritarian way of eating, it was useful for me to get support from people of like mind. But of course, you can certainly change your lifestyle without joining an online community.)

MY WEIGHT HAS NEVER BEEN THIS LOW

It took me just twelve months to lose eighty-one pounds and go from a BMI of 35.8 to 20.9 and go from 195.5 pounds to 114.5. My cholesterol went from 238 to 173, LDL from 146 to 108, triglycerides from 103 to 69, and glucose from 109 to 87.

My weight has never been this low, not even when I was in junior high school. Aches and pains are gone, my energy has greatly increased, and I feel absolutely wonderful! I now feel good in my skin now. This is not just about vanity; it is so much more than that. I can sit on the floor and play with my grandkids and not even know I have a body. I am no longer a slave to my appetite. I'm at peace with the knowledge that I'm doing what's best for my health, and I feel free! I am active and my body feels amazing. My social life has returned to normal, and I have an entirely new wardrobe to boot.

Has it been easy? No. But the small effort I have put forth is nothing in comparison to what I have gained. I have my life back!

What I have learned through this experience is that no food, along with the temporary pleasure it brings, is worth losing my health—nor is it worth the constant shame and discomfort I felt on a daily and even hourly basis. There are so many things we eat regularly that science has proven to be harmful to the body, and yet we keep on eating the same destructive foods over and over. I know this was the case with me. I have become fully convinced that I am a serious food addict. I used to pride myself on the fact that I was not food addicted. Boy, was I wrong!

It's shocking that I couldn't see the true depth of the problem, but as my husband always says, "Deception is so deceiving." I would eat plates and plates of food and continue eating way past satisfaction to the point that I would feel physical pain. Why would anyone keep eating when the food has lost it appeal and they are stuffed almost to the breaking point?

Most of the time I ate while not even being hungry and only because I wanted something tasty. And the main ingredients were always the same: foods with fat in copious amounts, and lots of salt and sugar; and of course anything made with white flour. When these items were in my diet, I had zero desire for vegetables or fruits of any kind. And interestingly, overeating and stuffing myself would happen only when I was eating the fat, salt, sugar, and white flour. I could eat doughnuts and white pasta until I felt like I was going to explode, but that never happened with green beans or apples. The healthy foods seem to be self-limiting.

Unfortunately for the addict, you cannot dabble with the

item of addiction. An alcoholic cannot have just one sip of alcohol. Pandora's box would then be opened. For the genuinely food-addicted individual, it's pretty much the same, and recent scientific evidence shows the brain chemistry involved in this reaction.[1] One bite of a fatty, gooey dessert or a little fettuccine Alfredo could set in motion a complete dive into gorging and overeating all of the wrong things. And from that point it sets in motion an avalanche that is very hard to stop. This is my experience as well as the experience of thousands of people who are food addicted. They do well eating healthfully until they taste something they know is a potential problem for them, and then an eating frenzy ensues.

This is also the problem with so-called "balanced" eating and the belief that anything in moderation is OK. For the addict, it is *not* OK. A little bite of this and a little bite of that may be fine for some, but for genuine food addicts it is virtually impossible to limit oneself when eating those highly palatable, fatty, sugary, salted foods. So what's the solution?

Well, if anyone had told me that when I started to eat healthfully, I would have to abstain (for the rest of my life) from most of what I ate, I would have told them there was no way I could make that commitment. And I didn't. So when I started my journey, I would schedule little cheat days or meals where I would eat all of my former favorite foods, believing that having a little something once a month was OK. This worked for a while (maybe for several months), and then it stopped working. I had awoken a sleeping giant! I started to find that the next day after my cheat days I wanted more of those foods, and I would yield. And then one cheat day would become two, and then three—you get the picture.

Moderation does not work for the addict, and it certainly didn't work for me. Abstinence was the only way. Is this easy? No, it's not. It's hard. Just like it's hard for the drug addict or the alcoholic to break with their addiction, it's hard for the food addict as well. It's hard to give up comfort foods you have eaten for decades. It's hard to be at family gatherings and be the only one not diving in to all the goodies there. It's hard to learn to enjoy foods you just do not like. It's hard. But on the other hand, it's hard being obese. It's hard hating to leave the house because of the shame you feel by being overweight, not to mention the fact that you're wearing your same old black fat "uniform." It's hard wearing long, dark pants and long-sleeved shirts in the height of the summer heat. It's hard to cover up all that fat, and most overweight individuals are acutely aware of this as they continue their daily ritual when getting dressed.

It's hard having high blood pressure, high cholesterol, and diabetes, and it's hard paying for the prescription meds necessary for these diseases caused by our overeating. It's hard playing and romping with your kids or grandkids when obese or overweight. It's hard living in a body that is in a perpetual state of discomfort due to encumbering fat. It's hard dying an early death from lifestyle diseases that are 99 percent preventable. It's hard.

When comparing the difficulty of changing my dietary habits to being overweight, I'd have to say the very hardest and most difficult thing for me would be having to live in an overweight body with all that entails, not only the physical problems but also the mental and emotional turmoil. My body is with me in everything I do every moment of every day. There is no escape from it. And as difficult as it is to abstain from unhealthful foods, living in an unhealthy body is far more difficult.

Living life unencumbered by overweight is a joy, as is living in control of my eating. I'm no longer driven by an overwhelming addiction and the uncontrollable urge to eat everything in sight. It's wonderful to be free.

Take every thought captive

Another simple thing but very powerful: I had to take my thoughts captive (2 Cor. 10:5) and control my mind from wandering and thinking about food. I have complete control over where my mind goes, and I should not let it wander wherever it wants to go. Daydreaming about fettuccine Alfredo and baby back ribs is not conducive to fighting temptation, and nothing positive comes of it. It creates desire. The more you think about a thing (food in this instance), the more fixated you become and the more you want it. The battle is truly in the mind, and it's like that with most non-food-related issues we deal with as well. If we can get a grip on our thought life, we can be free from so many of the things that bring us down spiritually. We need to be conscious of our thinking. Sometimes we're on autopilot and don't even realize we're having thoughts. This is one of those things that takes a lot of practice, but it can be done. Anything the Word instructs us to do is well within our reach.

Control your environment

I initially eliminated eating out because it was too tempting. I prepared all my own foods at home.

I kept any tempting foods out of the house. Since Mike was still eating unhealthily at the time I changed my diet, he prepared his own food. I did no cooking for him. I know this is not possible for everyone, but Mike was perfectly willing to eat out or cook his own meals, and this was a tremendous help and saved me from having to constantly fight off temptation. For mothers and fathers with kids at home, I fully understand how difficult it can be to have the responsibility of preparing meals for the entire household—making snacks all day and smelling and touching tempting food can be overwhelming. Serving your favorite junk food to others while denying yourself can be incredibly difficult. This is the time to sit down with your spouse and discuss your problem and the possible solutions.

One individual I know kept certain foods in a locked cabinet to which she didn't have a key because other family members wanted those junk foods in the house. Sometimes when one person changes, the entire household follows or at least improves some of their diet. Maybe your spouse can do the shopping and prepare some of the meals if you are the only one in the house choosing a healthy diet. Let your family know you need to clean out the pantry and fridge by removing the unhealthy and tempting items, or ask them to at least keep them out of your sight. The key thing here is identifying problems and weak points while working with your family members to find solutions.

Maybe your vulnerable time of the day is when the kids get off from school and arrive home wanting their snacks. Maybe it's when you have just walked in the door after work, and you're cranky and tired and in the habit of grabbing and eating the first thing you see. Many times you don't even fully enjoy it—it's just mindless eating. Come up with a plan ahead of time. Have the kids get their own snacks, which have been prepared by someone else earlier. Or better yet, maybe start preparing healthy snacks that the entire family can enjoy, and keep the junk out of the house. Have a plan for when the moment of temptation comes.

Maybe your weakness is when you're in the car, or specifically when you drive down a particular street. You could plan on taking a slightly different route or choose to bring something healthy to munch on. Maybe it's when you're at a ball game or sitting in front of the TV. Sometimes it's a specific television show, place, or sound that causes you to fixate on food for some unknown reason. I've muted television food commercials and consciously looked away many times. I've avoided situations, places, and events until I became stronger.

I've done whatever it takes with the wisdom God has given me to get the job done and secure my victory.

It may sound extreme, but we are bombarded constantly with images and odors and all sorts of things that are specifically designed to draw us in. Don't count on your strength or determination when faced with your usual temptation. Avoid it if you can and *flee*, or work on ways to circumvent the temptation if the situation is unavoidable.

The bottom line is God will make a way for you to make these changes in whatever circumstance of life you find yourself. He'll give you exactly what you need to succeed. Your needs may be different from mine, but the Lord will give you the wherewithal to accomplish what seems utterly impossible.

DETERMINING YOUR IDEAL WEIGHT

D R. JOEL FUHRMAN uses this formula to help you calculate your ideal weight, based on an average frame:

- For men: 105 pounds for the first 5 feet;
  5 pounds for each inch over 5 feet

- For women: 95 pounds for the first 5 feet;
  4 pounds for each inch over 5 feet

In my case, being just about 6 feet 3 inches tall, that's a total of 75 inches. So I start at 105 pounds for the first five feet (which equals 60 inches), then add 75 pounds (15 x 5) for a total of 180 pounds, which is pretty close to what I have weighed since dropping 95 pounds in less than eight months. It can vary a couple of pounds on either side, and I've definitely built up some more muscle, but this figure was exactly right for me as a medium-framed guy. If you're 5 feet 4 inches tall and female with a medium frame, your ideal weight would be 111 pounds (95 pounds for the first five feet plus 16 pounds (4 x 4) for the next 4 inches, for a total of 111 pounds).

For most of us, these figures seem incredibly low, and they're certainly less than the standard charts you see online. But even using those charts, most of us are overweight and many of us are obese. So calculate your ideal weight based on these guidelines, get on the scale, look to heaven, and say, "No excuses, Sir!"

RECOMMENDED RESOURCES

THERE ARE MANY websites and books that offer excellent advice for healthy living and eating. Listed here are the ones that Nancy and I found personally helpful or that adhere to the same guidelines we follow. There are some differences in the approaches of these doctors and nutritionists, but they are all plant based, which is so important.

WEBSITES

- Dr. Joel Fuhrman: https://www.drfuhrman.com/
- Dr. Michael Greger: http://nutritionfacts.org
- Dr. John McDoughall: https://www.drmcdougall.com
- Dr. Caldwell Esselstyn Jr.: http://www.dresselstyn.com/site/

RECIPES

- Dr. Joel Fuhrman, *Eat to Live Cookbook: 200 Delicious Nutrient-Rich Recipes for Fast and Sustained Weight Loss, Reversing Disease, and Lifelong Health* (New York: HarperOne, 2013)

- Ann Crile Esselstyn and Jane Esselstyn, *The Prevent and Reverse Heart Disease Cookbook: Over 125 Delicious, Life-Changing, Plant-Based Recipes* (New York: Avery, 2014)

- Dr. Fuhrman's Nutritarian Recipes Online: https://www.drfuhrman.com/lifestyle/recipes

- Cindy Marsch's Nutritarian Recipes blog: http://nutritarianrecipes.blogspot.com/

- Nutritarian recipes on Pinterest: https://www.pinterest.com/coco_gon_loco/nutritarian-recipes-for-everyday/

- *The Nutritarian Cooking Show With Jill Dalton*: https://www.youtube.com/channel/UCh2D2ss44sKdb6l7iGU7eLg https://nutritariancookingshow.com/

- Nutritarian Kids: http://nutritariankids.com/

- Motivated Mamas Nutritarian Recipe Share: http://www.motivatedmamas.net/2012/02/nutritarian-recipe-share.html

NOTES

CHAPTER 3: WHAT IF UNHEALTHY EATING IS SINFUL?

1. Joel Fuhrman, *Eat to Live* (New York: Little, Brown and Company, 2011), 15.

2. Roland Sturm and Kenneth B. Wells, "The Health Risks of Obesity: Worse Than Smoking, Drinking, or Poverty," RAND Health, accessed July 22, 2016, http://www.rand.org/pubs /research_briefs/RB4549.html.

3. Furhman, *Eat to Live*, 18.

4. Sarah Knapton, "Low-Fat Diets and Exercise Are Pointless for Losing Weight, Warns Surgical Expert," *The Telegraph*, June 9, 2016, accessed July 22, 2016, http://www.telegraph.co.uk /science/2016/06/09/low-fat-diets-and-exercise-are-pointless-for -losing-weight-warns/.

5. History.com Staff, "The 1918 Flu Pandemic," History.com (New York: A&E Networks, 2010), accessed July 22, 2016, http:// www.history.com/topics/1918-flu-pandemic.

6. H. D. M. Spence-Jones, ed., *The Pulpit Commentary: Proverbs* (New York: Funk & Wagnalls Company, 1909), 440.

7. Matthew Henry, *Matthew Henry's Commentary on the Whole Bible: Complete and Unabridged in One Volume* (Peabody, MA: Hendrickson Publishers, 1994), 1006.

8. Sturm and Wells, "The Health Risks of Obesity."

9. Ibid.

10. "Overweight and Obesity Statistics," The National Institute of Diabetes and Digestive and Kidney Diseases, accessed July 22, 2016, http://www.niddk.nih.gov/health-information/health -statistics/Pages/overweight-obesity-statistics.aspx.

11. Ibid.

12. Ibid.

13. Maggie Fox, "America's Obesity Epidemic Hits a New High," CNBC, June 7, 2016, accessed July 22, 2016, http://www.cnbc .com/2016/06/07/americas-obesity-epidemic-hits-a-new-high .html. As the article notes, obesity is "medically defined as

having a body mass index (BMI), a measure of height to weight, that's more than 30."

14. Furhman, *Eat to Live*, 146.

15. Sophie Borland, "Just Two Rashers of Bacon a Day Raises Your Risk of Cancer: Health Chiefs Put Processed Meat at Same Level as Cigarettes," *Daily Mail*, October 26, 2015, accessed July 22, 2016, http://www.dailymail.co.uk/health/article-3289821 /Bacon-burgers-sausages-big-cancer-threat-cigarettes-global -health-chiefs-declare.html#ixzz4FAeZa8l9.

16. Madlen Davies, "It's BETTER to Be Obese All Over Than Just Have a Beer Belly: Fat Around the Middle Can 'Double the Risk of Early Death,'" *Daily Mail*, November 2015, accessed July 22, 2016, http://www.dailymail.co.uk/health/article-3310633/It -s-BETTER-obese-just-beer-belly-Fat-middle-double-risk-early -death.html#ixzz42HyN3zs9.

17. Ben Spencer, "The World Now Has a Sweet Tooth: Soaring Sales of Soft Drinks and More Sugar in Foods Is Contributing to a 'Growing Crisis in Obesity, Diabetes and Heart Disease,'" *Daily Mail*, December 1, 2015, accessed July 22, 2016, http:// www.dailymail.co.uk/health/article-3341538/The-world-sweet -tooth-Soaring-sales-soft-drinks-sugar-foods-contributing -growing-crisis-obesity-diabetes-heart-disease.html.

18. Fiona Macrae, "Cancer ISN'T All in Your Genes: Up to 90% of Cases 'Could Be Wiped Out by Avoiding Triggers Caused by Our Unhealthy Lifestyles,'" *Daily Mail*, December 16, 2015, accessed July 22, 2016, http://www.dailymail.co.uk/health/ article-3362965/How-cancer-ISN-T-genes-90-cancer-wiped -avoiding-triggers-caused-unhealthy-lifestyles .html#ixzz42I03KNNO.

19. Madlen Davies, "Revealed, Your Body on Sugar: From Weak- ening the Immune System to Triggering Thrush, This Terrifying Tool Reveals Exactly How the White Stuff Harms Our Health," *Daily Mail*, March 24, 2016, accessed July 22, 2016, http://www .dailymail.co.uk/health/article-3507655/Revealed-body-sugar -weakening-immune-triggering-thrush-terrifying-tool-reveals -exactly-white-stuff-harms-health.html#ixzz43tDqYIen.

20. Joel Furhman, "The American Diet Is Shortening Our Chil- dren's Lives," *Food & Health With Timi Gustafson, R.D.* (blog), accessed August 22, 2016, http://www.timigustafson.com/2014 /american-diet-shortening-childrens-lives/; see also "Children's

Health" at http://www.drfuhrman.com/library/childrens
_longevity.aspx.

21. W. Arndt, F. W. Danker, and W. Bauer, *A Greek-English Lexicon of the New Testament and Other Early Christian Literature*, 3rd ed. (Chicago: University of Chicago Press, 2000), 274.

22. F. F. Bruce, *The Epistle to the Galatians: A Commentary on the Greek Text* (Grand Rapids, MI: W.B. Eerdmans Pub. Co., 1982), 255.

CHAPTER 5: TOO FAT TO FLY

1. Jackie MacMullan, "How Draymond Green and Kevin Love Wage War—on Their Weight," ESPN, June 12, 2016, accessed July 22, 2016, http://espn.go.com/nba/story/_/id/16080927/how-draymond-green-kevin-love-wage-war-their-weight.

2. Ibid.

3. Ibid.

CHAPTER 6: ANTI-FAT CREAM AND THE MAGIC ENERGY PILL

1. For a fascinating, related story, see Paul Offit, "The Vitamin Myth: Why We Think We Need Supplements," *The Atlantic*, July 19, 2013, accessed July 22, 2016, http://www.theatlantic.com/health/archive/2013/07/the-vitamin-myth-why-we-think-we-need-supplements/277947/.

CHAPTER 7: MY PLAN WAS NOT WORKING

1. Joel Fuhrman, *The End of Dieting* (New York: HarperCollins, 2014); Joel Furhman, *Eat to Live*.

CHAPTER 8: HOW MY RADICAL TRANSFORMATION BEGAN

1. "Description of High Blood Pressure," National Heart, Lung and Blood Institute, September 10, 2015, accessed September 6, 2016, http://www.nhlbi.nih.gov/health/health-topics/topics/hbp.

2. Ibid.

CHAPTER 9: BREAKING THE FOOD ADDICTIONS AND REPROGRAMMING MY MIND

1. For example, Dr. Joel Furhman's *Eat to Live Cookbook*.

2. Joel Fuhrman, *The End of Dieting*, 22–23.

3. Ibid.

4. Connecticut College Staff, "Student-Faculty Research [at a Connecticut college] Suggests Oreos Can Be Compared to Drugs of Abuse in Lab Rats," Connecticut College, October 15, 2013, accessed July 23, 2016, https://www.conncoll.edu/news/news-archive/2013/student-faculty-research-suggests-oreos-can-be-compared-to-drugs-of-abuse-in-lab-rats.html#.VtE2m5wrJ1g.

5. Ibid.

6. Ibid.

7. Furhman, *Eat to Live*, 216; Fuhrman, *The End of Dieting*, 153–158.

CHAPTER 12: THE ESAU MENTALITY IS DEADLY

1. Thomas Brooks, *The Select Works of Thomas Brooks* (London: L. B. Seely and Son), 317, viewed at GoogleBooks.

2. The letters "kh" represent the equivalent of "ch" in the Scottish word "loch."

3. For its varied usages in the Old Testament, see Andrew Hill, "*acharit*," in the *New International Dictionary of Old Testament Theology and Exegesis (NIDOTTE)*, vol. 1 (Grand Rapids, MI: Zondervan, 1997), 361–362, with references to other, more complete treatments of the word on page 362. In Exodus 33:23 the related word *'achôr* occurs in a plural form with reference to God's "back"; in Ezekiel 8:16 it refers to the backs of people.

4. Note Isaiah 46:10, "I make known the end from the beginning" (NIV), where the word for end is *'acharit*, derived from the word for "that which comes after; back," and the word for beginning is *re'šit*, derived from the word for "head."

5. I have translated this literally to bring out the force of the original; for the Hebrew word *mûsar*, meaning "discipline; instruction," see Eugene H. Merrill, "*ysr*," in the *New International Dictionary of Old Testament Theology and Exegesis (NIDOTTE)*, vol. 2 (Grand Rapids, MI: Zondervan, 1997), 479–82, especially 480–81.

CHAPTER 13: EXCUSES ARE FOR WIMPS

1. I have written about my increased call for preachers, teachers, and Bible translators to stop using the name James instead of Jacob in reference to Jesus's disciple. The Greek uses *Jacob* throughout the New Testament. For more on this, see Michael Brown, "Recovering the Lost Letter of Jacob," *Charisma News*, March 11, 2013, accessed July 25, 2016, http://www .charismanews.com/opinion/38591-recovering-the-lost-letter-of -jacob.

2. Today she would recommend a "nutritarian" diet, as per Dr. Fuhrman; see his book *The End of Diabetes*.

CHAPTER 14: HOLINESS PRINCIPLES FOR WHOLESOME EATING

1. D. A. Carson, "Matthew," *The Expositor's Bible Commentary*, vol. 7, gen. ed. F. E. Gaebelein (Grand Rapids, MI: Zondervan, 1984), 151.

2. Thomas Brooks, *The Select Works of Thomas Brooks* (London: L.B. Seely and Son), 317, viewed at GoogleBooks.

3. Charles H. Spurgeon, *Morning by Morning* (Peabody, MA: Hendrickson Publishers, 2006), 151.

CHAPTER 15: TEN RECOMMENDATIONS FOR A HEALTHY LIFESTYLE

1. Joel Fuhrman, "Study on 'The Biggest Loser' Contestants: The Body Adapts to Regain Lost Weight," Dr. Fuhrman Online, accessed July 25, 2016, http://tinyurl.com/zfkvqjs.

2. For a very helpful article on this, see Dr. Joel Fuhrman, "The Dangers of Weight Cycling (Yo-Yo Dieting)," Dr. Fuhrman Online, accessed September 6, 2016, http://www.drfuhrman .com/library/dangers-yo-yo-dieting.aspx.

3. Fuhrman, "Study on 'The Biggest Loser' Contestants: The Body Adapts to Regain Lost Weight."

4. "Dunkin' Donuts Chocolate Glazed Cake Donut," CalorieKing, accessed July 25, 2016, http://www.calorieking.com/foods /calories-in-donuts-chocolate-glazed-cake-donut_f -ZmlkPTU2Mjg2.html.

5. "Java Chip Frappuccino Blended Coffee," Starbucks, accessed July 25, 2016, http://www.starbucks.com/menu/drinks/frappuccino-blended-beverages/java-chip-frappuccino-blended-beverage#size=11002667&milk=67&whip=125.

6. "Saturated Fats," American Heart Association, accessed July 25, 2016, http://www.heart.org/HEARTORG/HealthyLiving/HealthyEating/Nutrition/Saturated-Fats_UCM_301110_Article.jsp#.Vy1ghjArI2w.

7. See Kevin Gianni's interview with Dr. Joel Furhman, "Why [You're] Addicted to Certain Foods with Dr. Joel Fuhrman #658," Renegade Health, accessed July 25, 2016, https://www.youtube.com/watch?v=eyMBOr0Nq1M._

8. Neal Barnard, *Breaking the Food Seduction: The Hidden Reasons Behind Food Cravings—and 7 Steps to End Them Naturally* (New York: St. Martin's Press, 2003).

9. "Dr. Fuhrman: Stop Food Addiction, Lose Weight, True Hunger vs Toxic Hunger," ANewDayANewMe, accessed July 25, 2016, http://www.anewdayanewme.com/dr-fuhrman-stop-food-addiction-lose-weight-true-hunger-vs-toxic-hunger/; "Hungry? True Hunger Versus Toxic Hunger," Dr. Fuhrman, accessed September 8, 2016, https://www.drfuhrman.com/learn/library/articles/25/hungry-true-hunger-versus-toxic-hunger.

APPENDIX A: NANCY'S STORY

1. See, e.g., Kris Gunnars, "How Sugar Hijacks Your Brain and Makes You Addicted," Authority Nutrition, accessed September 6, 2016, https://authoritynutrition.com/how-sugar-makes-you-addicted/.

CONNECT WITH US!

CHARISMA HOUSE

(Spiritual Growth)

Facebook.com/CharismaHouse

@CharismaHouse

Instagram.com/CharismaHouseBooks

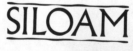

SILOAM

(Health)

Pinterest.com/CharismaHouse

REALMS

(Fiction)

Facebook.com/RealmsFiction